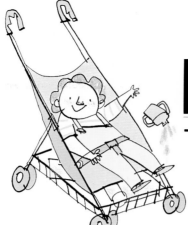

BIRTH TO FIVE

GW00702247

Contents

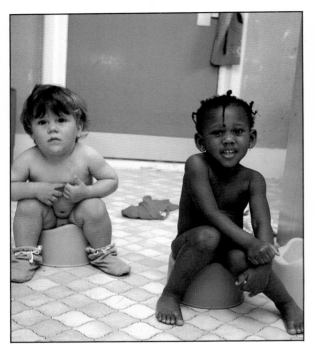

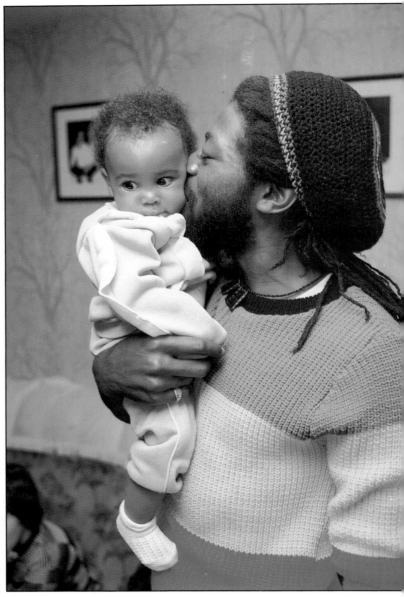

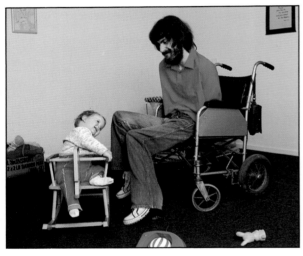

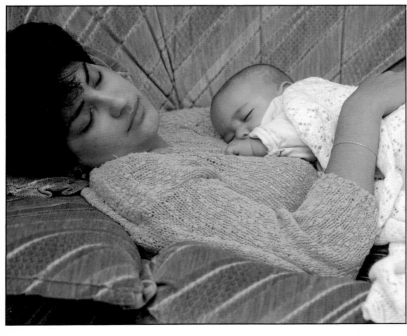

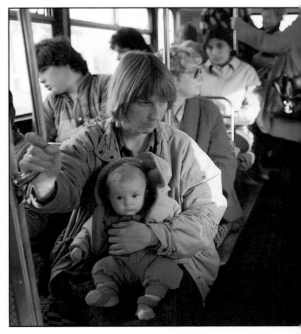

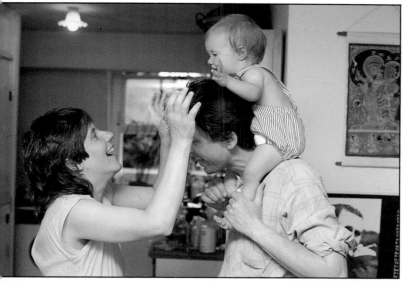

This book

No-one needs a book to tell them what's good about being a parent. Parents turn to books when they need information, when they're worried, when they've got questions or worries, small or large. This is a book you can turn to.

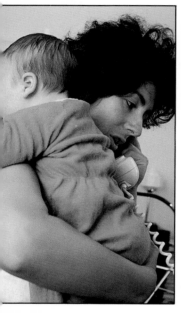

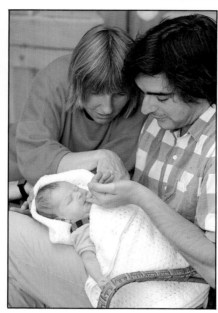

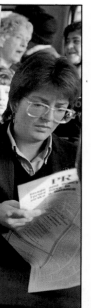

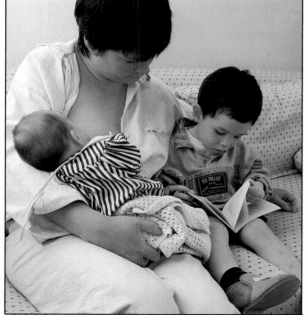

1. Babies

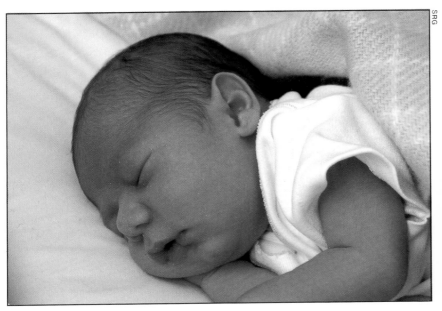

"It's great. She's great. But it's 24 hours a day. And you don't think it's great when you're changing a nappy at four in the morning, or when she's been crying non-stop for an hour."

(A father) "I didn't think I'd feel the way I do about her. Sometimes I look at her when she's sleeping, you know, and I have to put my face down next to hers, just to check she's breathing."

"There was none of this love at first sight. It was a long time before I came to love him. I can say that now, but at the time I couldn't tell anybody. I thought there was something wrong with me. There was all that work, and feeling rough myself, and because I didn't have this overwhelming feeling for him, none of it made much sense. But oh yes, after three or four months or so of all that, yes, it came right then."

"Because we nearly lost him, and I saw what it would be like if we *had* lost him, I can cope with anything now, it doesn't matter how hard it is."

"There are so many people telling you what to do and how to do it, you get to think there's a right way and a wrong way, and mostly you seem to be doing it the wrong way. It's not true. After all, it's your baby, and it's for you to decide. You have to sort out your own way of doing things. Other people can only tell you so much."

"Doctors and health visitors look at you as if to say you're worrying over nothing, but it's not nothing, is it? It's your whole world – or that's what it feels like at the time. Other mothers understand, the other mothers I meet who've got first babies."

(A father) "Sure, I want to help. And when I'm at home, I *do* help as much as I can. But that's not much for me, is it? Being a father isn't just 'helping'. It's difficult, because so much goes on when I'm not at home, and then it's easy for Ann to say, you know, 'You're doing that wrong' or 'Let me do that'."

"At first, I think he thought it would be dead easy for him. You know, he thought he'd come home, and there'd be supper on the table, and the baby clean and smiling, and me clean and smiling . . . Now he comes home and *he* gets supper, and maybe after an hour or so I *am* clean, or smiling – probably not both."

Coping with it all

For some parents, the first months with a new baby are happy and easy. For some, they are happy but hard. For some, they are just hard.

Coping with it all doesn't mean getting everything done. It means doing what you can and feeling all right about leaving the rest. It means caring for yourself as well as for your baby. It means finding a way of living happily through a tiring, maybe difficult time.

Think about:

○ Ways of cutting down the work. Don't do what you don't have to do. You and your baby are more important than the housework. Other people have to understand that.

○ Ways of sharing the work, with your partner or anybody you can find. Accept offers of help, and if no-one offers, ask. Asking for help doesn't mean you're a failure.

○ Organising life your way. There are no rules about when, for example, you should bath your baby, and no rule that says babies have to be bathed every day. Do things the way that suits you and your baby.

○ Making some time for yourself, to rest, relax, sleep, eat a proper meal, but also to do whatever you want to do.

○ Making time to be with your partner, or whoever you can relax and talk with.

○ Taking time – even just odd moments – to do *nothing* but enjoy your baby.

○ And taking each day as it comes.

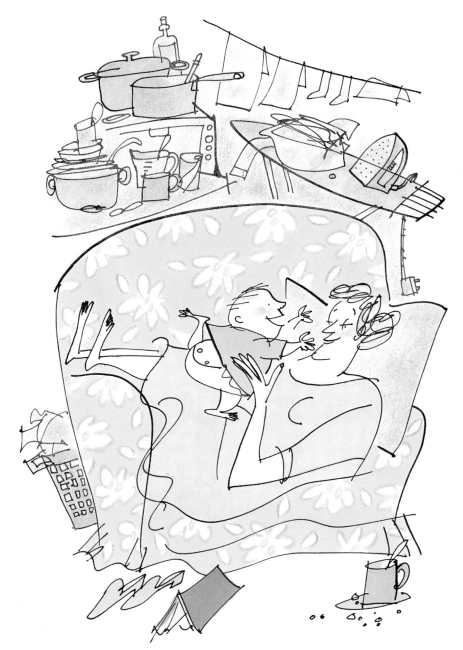

All parents with small babies need help and support. You can't cope alone, not all the time. You need people around you, and from time to time, you will probably need professional help too. Look at Chapter 6 for information about where to find help and support.

If you're bringing up your baby alone, see page 38. If you're coping with a second baby, see pages 38-9.

"People talk about babies the same way as all the books and adverts talk about babies. So it feels like babies aren't supposed to yell, and you're not supposed to be exhausted, and you never run out of nappies, and your breasts don't leak and stain the one clean sweater you've got, and the baby never sicks up on your shoulder... and all those things that happen every day to me. And if you're not careful, you end up feeling guilty because you're not some kind of television super-mum."

"I don't think anybody can tell you beforehand how much a baby changes your life. If they do try to tell you, you don't believe them. I know it's taken me a long time to accept that everything is different now. It was when I stopped trying to go on exactly like before, trying so hard I wore myself out, that was when it got better."

Breast feeding

"I suppose I'd thought that I'd just put her to my breast and that would be it. I hadn't thought of it as something I might have to learn about and practise. So it came as a bit of a shock that the first weeks were really quite tough. But I was determined I was going to do it, and yes, it's lovely now."

"I was quite tense at first. I worried whether I was doing it right, and whether I was giving her enough, and I was feeling a bit weepy anyway. You need to find somebody to help and give you confidence. Maybe I was lucky, but my midwife was fantastic. And once I'd got her help, I just relaxed about the whole thing."

Quite a lot of first-time mothers find the early weeks of breast feeding hard. Hold on to the the fact that breast feeding is best for your baby. Keep going, get help if you need it, and have confidence. If you can learn how to do it and sort out any problems, breast feeding will be good for you too – convenient, cheap, and a real pleasure.

THE ADVANTAGES OF BREAST FEEDING

○ Breast milk is the only food designed and meant for your baby. It contains the nutrients your baby needs for health and development. It is easily digested. It is less likely to cause stomach upsets or diarrhoea. It helps avoid constipation.

○ Breast milk also contains antibodies and other protective factors which help protect your baby against infections. The formula milk used for bottle feeding doesn't contain these antibodies.

○ There is some evidence to show that breast fed babies are less likely to get allergies.

○ If your baby was born prematurely, breast feeding is especially important.

○ Breast feeding is very practical. There is no cost. There's no preparation. The milk is always there when needed.

○ Breast feeding can help you to get your shape back more quickly.

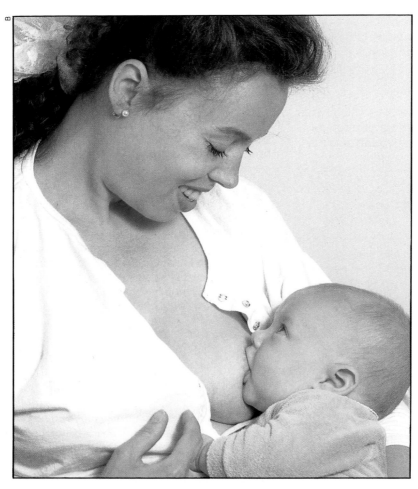

How breast feeding works

Understanding how breast feeding works can help you make it work.

Your milk supply   Your breasts produce milk in answer to your baby feeding at your breast. The more your baby feeds, the more milk you produce. So, if you let your baby feed whenever a feed is wanted, you should produce the amount of milk your baby needs. If you are ever worried that you haven't got enough milk, feeding your baby will be at least part of the answer. Feeding more often will increase your milk supply.

You produce less milk when you are tired and low on energy. So resting and eating well are also important. You need to drink plenty too. A rest and something to eat in the afternoon will help if your baby is one of the many who want to feed a lot in the evening.

The 'let-down' reflex   Your baby's feeding also causes the 'let-down' of the milk. That is, it makes the milk flow down and gather behind the nipple. Sometimes this happens even before your baby starts to feed, maybe when you hear your baby cry. In the early weeks, milk may start to leak from your breasts.

The let-down reflex is important. Without it, your baby can't get your milk. For the reflex to work, your baby has to be in the right position at your breast (see 'Your baby's position' opposite). And you need to be fairly relaxed. Stress, worry, exhaustion, pain, even embarrassment can all stop the let-down reflex working. If you're anxious and under stress, it may not seem very helpful to be told to stop worrying and relax. But it's probably what you need to do, if you can only find a way of doing it. Look at 'Coping with it all' on page 5. And if you have any worry or problem over feeding, ask for help (see 'Help with breast feeding,' page 9).

How your baby feeds   Unlike the teat on a bottle, there's no milk in the nipple itself. Once the milk has been 'let down', it gathers *behind* the nipple and areola (the dark area around the nipple). So a baby who only sucks on the nipple doesn't get much milk. To make the milk flow out, your baby's mouth needs to be wide open and his or her lips and gums have to press against the area *around* the nipple. This is why your baby's position at your breast is so important.

Finding the right position

Your position   Make yourself comfortable. You need to be able to hold your baby close to your breast without strain, and for some time. Try different chairs and different ways of sitting. Try a pillow to raise your baby higher. Try lying down on your side with your baby up against you. Find what's best for you.

Later, you won't have to think about what position you're in. You'll be able to feed almost however and wherever you want to.

Your baby's position   Hold your baby close and turned towards you, so his or her chest (not side) is against you.

Your baby needs to take your nipple with a wide-open mouth, taking in not just the nipple but also much of the area around – more *below* than above. Your baby's chin should be touching your breast.

You can make your baby turn towards your breast by gently rubbing your nipple against your baby's cheek.

How often, how long?

Some babies settle into a pattern of feeding quite quickly. Others take longer. In the early weeks, you may find that feeds are sometimes long, sometimes short, sometimes close together, sometimes further apart. Just try to follow what your baby tells you. Feed when your baby asks to be fed, and for as long as your baby wants.

Once you've put your baby to your breast, let the feed go on until your baby wants to stop. Then, either straight away or after a pause, offer the other breast to see if your baby wants more. If you swap from one breast to the other before your baby is ready, you may only be giving the 'foremilk' from each breast. The 'hindmilk' which comes later, contains the calories your baby needs.

Allow your baby to decide when he or she has had enough. Both breasts won't always be wanted at each feed. Your baby will show when he or she has finished by either letting go of your breast or falling asleep. Try to remember to start each feed on alternate breasts.

If you feed as often and for as long as your baby wants, you will produce plenty of milk and give your baby what he or she needs. While your baby is very young, this may mean quite lengthy feeds. But if you've got your baby in the right position at your breast, you shouldn't become sore. And feeds won't go on like this for ever. If you feel at first that you are doing nothing but feeding, try to remember that that's good for your baby now, and that it will become easier for you later.

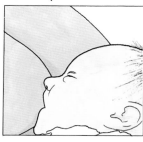

Your baby needs to feed with a wide-open mouth, taking in the nipple and also much of the area around. ▼

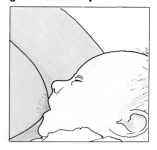

If your baby sucks on the nipple alone he or she won't get much milk. ▼

How much is enough?

Since it's impossible to see how much milk a baby is taking from the breast, mothers often worry whether they are giving enough. You can be sure you are giving enough milk if your baby –

– is generally gaining weight. Some babies gain weight steadily. Other perfectly healthy babies gain little or no weight one week, then feed more often and make up for it over the next week or two. It is overall weight gain that's important. (See page 23 for weight checks.)

– has at least six really wet nappies a day (and is having nothing but breast milk).

If, at any time during the first two to three months, your baby is feeding less than five to six times in 24 hours, is gaining weight only slowly, or is very sleepy and feeding poorly, talk to your midwife or health visitor.

Hunger, or thirst?

Breast milk is drink and food in one. So whether your baby is crying from hunger or thirst, breast feeding is usually the answer. There is no need to give your baby drinks of water, even in a very hot climate.

BREASTFEEDING PROBLEMS

Painful feeding   Some women find breast feeding hurts during the first week or two. Your milk supply has to settle down, and your nipples have to grow used to your baby's sucking. After this, if feeding still hurts, it's a sign that your baby's position is wrong. If you can't get the position right yourself, ask for help.

Feeding restlessly   If your baby is restless at the breast and doesn't seem satisfied by feeds, it may be that he or she is sucking on the nipple alone and so isn't getting enough milk. Check that your baby is in the right position at your breast. Ask for help if you need to.

Engorged (swollen) breasts   The answer is to feed. If feeding is difficult for some reason, ask for help. To ease the swelling, try a hot bath, or bathing your breasts with warm water. Smooth out some milk with your fingers, stroking gently downwards towards the nipple. Or try a facecloth, wrung out in very cold water, held against your breast. Check your bra is not too tight.

Sore or cracked nipples
After the first two weeks of feeding, if your baby is in the right position at your breast, feeding shouldn't hurt even if your nipples *are* sore or cracked. So check your baby's position and ask for help if you need it.

Keep your nipples clean and dry. Change breastpads often. Let the air get to your nipples as much as possible. Try sleeping topless, if it's warm enough, with a towel under you if you are leaking milk.

If none of this works, you could try nipple shields from the chemist. These fit over your nipples like teats. Your baby sucks on the shield not your nipple. But don't use shields for more than a day or so. They may reduce your milk supply.

Sometimes sore nipples are caused by *thrush* in a baby's mouth. Thrush is an infection that causes small white patches, which rub off to show

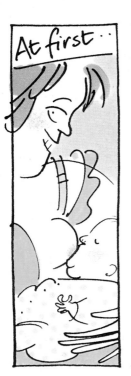 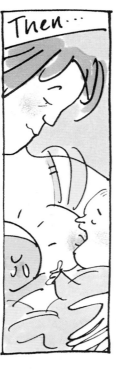 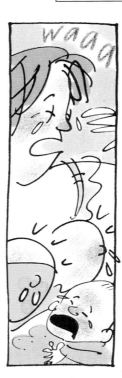 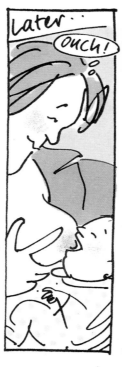 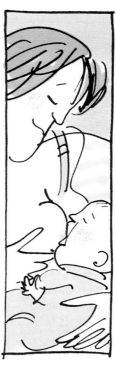 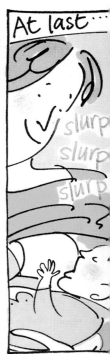

raw, red skin underneath. it can be easily treated, but the breast has to be treated as well. If you think your baby has thrush, see your doctor.

Lumpy, tender breasts can be caused by blocked ducts. Milk builds up because the ducts aren't being emptied properly. Check that your bra isn't too tight and that nothing is pressing into your breast as you feed (your bra, or arm, for example).

A good feed on the blocked breast will help. As you feed, smooth the milk away from the blockage towards your nipple. If this doesn't work, ask for help. If left untreated, blocked ducts can lead to mastitis.

Mastitis Your breast will be inflamed. There will be a patch that is flushed and hot. Don't stop feeding because it will help to get your milk moving. Try feeding in different positions to empty different parts of the breast. Get lots of rest. Go to bed if you can. Bathe your breast in warm water, or try a hot or cold facecloth, held against your breast.

Mastitis can become an infection, making you feel unwell, as though you've got flu. If you feel like this, see, or call, your doctor. You will probably need an antibiotic. Your doctor can prescribe one which is safe to take while breast feeding.

HELP WITH BREAST FEEDING

You can get help and advice from:

○ your community midwife, health visitor or doctor

○ a breastfeeding counsellor or support group. Contact your local branch of the National Childbirth Trust, La Leche League, or Association of Breastfeeding Mothers (addresses on page 94). These organisations give help and support through other mothers with experience of breast feeding.

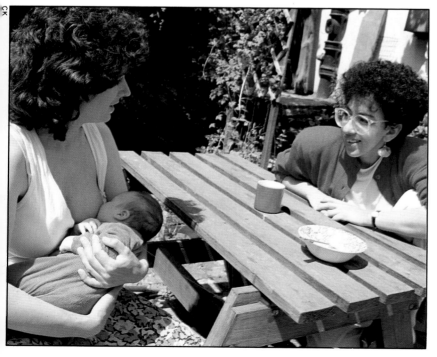

Coping with breast feeding

Breast feeding is lovely when it goes well. But if it doesn't go well, it can cause a lot of stress and upset. The stress then affects the feeding, and things go from bad to worse. Other kinds of stress, or just general worry and tiredness, can also affect breast feeding. You stand a much better chance of breast feeding successfully if you can relax and care for yourself.

○ If you have any worries or problems to do with feeding, ask for help. (See 'Help with breast feeding', opposite.) The right sort of support can make all the difference.

○ Try to keep on top of things – and when you're not on top, try not to mind. Look at 'Coping with it all' on page 5.

○ Breast feeding uses energy and you may feel hungrier than usual. Eat as you feel you need to. It will help to keep you going and keep your milk supply up. You may be thirsty too, and to produce milk, you need to take fluids. Drinking milk is a quick way of getting both the fluid and the extra calories you need. You may want to settle down for a breast feed with a drink and some food beside you.

○ Feeding when your baby wants to be fed is good for your baby but may make life tough for you. You may feel constantly in demand. Try to accept it: the feeling does go as your baby settles into a pattern of feeding. Feeding's important, and for a time other things will have to take second place. Don't sit with your baby at your breast looking at the dirty dishes or the dust. Try to make the most of a bit of peace and quiet.

○ Some women find breast feeding in front of others awkward and embarrassing. Most get used to it in time, and find ways of doing it discreetly. But you don't have to breast feed in public if you don't want to. It's usually possible to go into another room. Many places such as large shops now provide places for mothers to feed. If not, ask whether there is somewhere you could feed in private.

○ Once you've got breast feeding going, you may want to express some milk for someone else to give to your baby in a bottle. If you're feeling worn down and exhausted, it can be a relief if one feed in a day is someone else's responsibility. And it can give a lot of pleasure to your partner, or maybe a grandparent. The odd feed of expressed milk from a bottle won't affect your baby's breast feeding. In fact, if you can get your baby used to the bottle, it can be an advantage later when you want to leave your baby with someone else.

Your midwife or health visitor will show you how to express. You can then store the milk in a sterilised, capped bottle in the fridge. (Don't keep it for longer than 24 hours.) You can also freeze breast milk if you want to keep it for a few weeks. When you want to use it, put it in the fridge until completely defrosted.

Combining breast and bottle

If you are worried that you are not producing enough milk for your baby, giving the odd bottle of formula milk is *not* the answer. it will mean that you produce less milk, not more. Breast feeding more often will increase your milk supply.

But if you are going back to work, you will probably need to combine breast and bottle feeds. The bottle feeds might be expressed breast milk, or formula milk. Some women can express enough milk to cover the time when they are away. Ask you health visitor or contact one of the breastfeeding organisations for advice. If you use formula milk, you can still carry on with, say, morning and evening breast feeds. If you make this a regular thing, your milk supply should adjust.

Try to get your baby used to taking a bottle before you go back to work.

Changing from breast to bottle

If, for whatever reason, you decide to change from breast to bottle feeding, it's best if you can do it gradually. Change one feed a day at first, then two, and so on. Try to choose the feed when you think you stand the best chance of success. For example, it's probably best not to give the first bottle feeds at times when your baby is tired.

It may help if someone other than you gives the first bottle feeds. Your baby is not then near your breast, smelling and expecting breast milk.

You can buy bottles which have more 'breast-like' teats. You can also buy the teats separately. These may be the answer if your baby isn't taking to the bottle.

Not all babies take to the bottle easily. Many mothers have very mixed feelings about changing to the bottle, especially if they badly wanted to breast feed. If your baby then doesn't seem to like the bottle, the changeover can be upsetting. Don't feel guilty. Your baby will take to bottle feeding eventually, and it is a perfectly good way of feeding a baby.

If, on the other hand, you have started giving the odd bottle but then decide you want to go back to full breast feeding, you can do it if you want to. If your baby is under three weeks old, you can probably cut out bottles all at once. If your baby is older, or is having a lot of bottles, cut out the bottle feeding over a few days. If you breast feed your baby often, and for longer, your milk supply will increase. For a day or two, you will have to feed a lot, but this won't go on for long. Feeds will space out again once your milk supply has increased.

Wind –
and what may come with it

After a feed, you may want to see if your baby has any wind to come up. Hold your baby against your shoulder or propped forward a bit on your lap and gently rub his or her back. You don't have to do this, although often it's a nice way of being close after a feed. Some babies seem 'windier' than others. If you happen to have a 'windy' baby, it's a good idea. (For information about **colic** see page 17.)

Some babies also sick up more than others. (Sicking up milk during or just after a feed is called 'possetting'.) It's not unusual for a baby to sick up quite a bit. Have a cloth handy to mop up. If your baby brings back a lot of milk, remember he or she is likely to be hungry again quite quickly. If this happens often, if your baby is frequently or violently sick, or if you are worried for any other reason, see your health visitor or doctor.

Vitamins

You will probably be advised to give your baby vitamin drops from the age of six months. Sometimes they are suggested earlier. The drops contain the vitamins A, C and D.

Go on giving five drops a day until your child is at least two years old. By this age, many children are getting the vitamins they need from the food they eat and don't need extra. But if your child doesn't eat a wide range of foods, then it is probably best to go on with the drops until the age of five.

Vitamin D, which is important for strong bones, is different from other vitamins. It is found in some foods but it is also made by the body as a result of sunlight on bare skin. So children who are indoors a lot may not get enough of it. If you think your child may be short of vitamin D, carry on giving vitamin drops until he or she is five.

Don't give any other vitamin supplements (such as cod liver oil) in addition to the drops. Too much of some vitamins is as harmful as not enough.

You can get vitamin drops at most child health clinics. See 'Help with national health service costs', page 92 to check whether you can claim free vitamins.

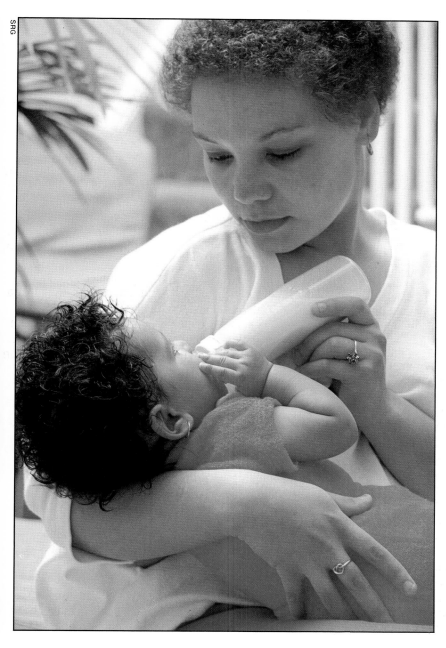

Bottle feeding

(A father) **"I wouldn't have missed it. When he was small, those feeds brought us close. It was how we got to know each other."**

Early on, if the feeds weren't going well, I'd think, well, perhaps I'd better try a different kind of milk, or a different bottle, or a different teat, or whatever. But it's the same as doing anything for the first time. It's a while before you know what you're doing, and then you settle down and start to enjoy it."

Get well organised for bottle feeding so that you can enjoy it. In time, you'll find your own routine for preparing feeds and sterilising.

You need

at least six bottles and teats   There are different kinds. Ask your midwife, health visitor or other mothers if you want advice on what to buy. You may be able to get secondhand bottles (say, from a friend) and buy new teats, but make sure the bottles are in good condition. If they've been heavily used and the plastic scratched, you won't be able to sterilise them properly.

a supply of baby milk (formula milk). Again, there are lots of different brands and you may want advice on which to choose. Most formula milks are made from cow's milk, specially treated to make it suitable for babies. If there's a strong history of allergies in your family, a soya formula might be recommended.

You may be able to buy baby milk cheaper at your clinic than in the shops.

See page 92 'Help with national health service costs', to check whether you can claim free or low-price milk for your baby.

sterilising equipment (see page 12).

Making up feeds

⬤ To make up the milk, follow the instructions on the tin or packet. It's important to follow them exactly. Don't add extra powder, or anything else, to make a 'stronger' feed. And don't add sugar.

⬤ You'll gradually learn how much milk to make up. The instructions on the tin or packet will guide you. As a guide, a baby needs about 150ml of milk per 1kg body weight (2½oz per 1lb) every 24 hours.

⬤ You can, if you want, make up a day's feeds in advance and store the capped bottles in the fridge. This saves time, and means you don't have to make your baby wait while you make up a feed. Don't keep the made-up milk for longer than 24 hours. Shake the bottle well before you use it.

Sterilising

Sterilising bottles and teats protects your baby against infection. You can sterilise either by using chemical sterilising tablets or liquid, or by using a microwave bottle steriliser. (Microwave ovens are *only* suitable for sterilising if you have a special microwave bottle steriliser.)

Chemical sterilising

You can buy complete sterilising units in the shops, or you can use a plastic bucket with a lid.

1. Wash the bottles and teats thoroughly, using washing-up liquid. Get rid of every trace of milk, squirting water through the teats and using a bottle brush for the bottles.

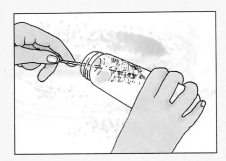

2. Rinse in clean water, then immerse everything in sterilising solution. To make up the solution, follow the instructions which come with the sterilising tablets or liquid. Leave the bottles and teats in the solution for the time given in the instructions. If you're using a bucket, keep everything under the water by putting a plate on top. Make sure there aren't any air bubbles inside the bottles.

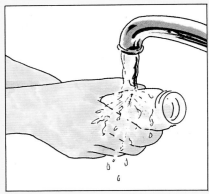

3. When you take the bottles and teats out to make up feeds, don't rinse them with tap water because you will make them unsterile again. If you want to rinse off the sterilising solution, use boiled cooled water.

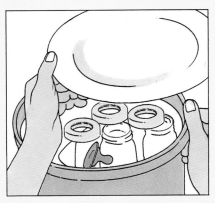

Feeding

○ You can warm the bottle before a feed by standing it in some hot water. Test the temperature of the milk by squirting some onto your wrist. Some babies don't mind cold milk, others like it warmed. Don't keep the milk warm for more than an hour before a feed: germs breed in the warmth.

It is unsafe to use a microwave oven for warming a bottle of milk. The milk continues to heat for a time after you take it out of the microwave, yet the outside of the bottle feels cold.

○ Get yourself comfortable so you can cuddle your baby close as you feed. Give your baby time, and let him or her take as much milk as he or she wants. Some babies take some milk, drop off to sleep, then wake up for more. Be patient. At the end of a feed, throw away any left-over milk.

○ As you feed, keep the bottle tilted so the teat is always full of milk. Otherwise your baby will be taking in air.

○ If the teat flattens while you are feeding, pull gently on the bottle to release the vacuum. If the teat blocks, start again with another sterile teat.

○ Teats come in all sorts of shapes and with different hole sizes. You may need to experiment to find the right teat and hole size for your baby. If the hole is too small, your baby will suck and suck without getting enough milk. If it's too big, your baby will get too much too quickly and probably spit and splutter or bring the feed back. A small teat hole can be made larger with a red-hot needle.

○ Never prop up a bottle and leave your baby to feed alone, in case of choking.

○ Don't add solids to bottle feeds as this can cause choking.

Thirst

If you think your baby is more thirsty than hungry, perhaps because the weather is hot, try a bottle of water, boiled first then cooled.

If you want help or advice on bottle feeding, talk to your midwife or health visitor, or to other mothers with experience of bottle feeding.

Starting solid food

"With your first baby, you worry about what you give them, and how much, and whether they'll like it. But with your second, it's much more like they have to fit in with the rest of the family, and you don't think about it so much. They take what's going, and they do it for themselves really."

"I think a lot of fuss is made about it and you can get to think it's more complicated than it really is. Maybe if you start when your baby is very young, maybe then you do have to be a bit careful. But when your baby's ready for it, she tells you what she wants. With mine, if she takes something and likes it, that's fine. And if she spits something out, I give that a rest for a while."

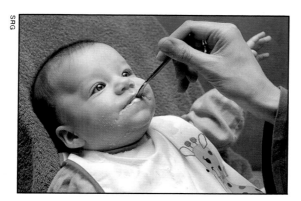

When to start

"I think there's a lot of pressure on you to stop the breast feeding and, you know, get onto something a bit more substantial. People are always sort of pushing you on to the next stage. It's hard to know what's best when people are saying to you, 'Isn't she weaned yet?' and 'Have you tried this, have you tried that?' "

Very few babies need solid food before they are four months old and almost all should have started some solid food by about six months. Most babies are ready to start when they are about four months old.

How can you tell when your baby is ready?
Give solid foods a try when your baby–
- still seems hungry after finishing a good milk feed and you've tried giving more milk.
- starts to demand feeds more often.
- maybe, after sleeping through the night, starts waking again to be fed.
- seems more restless than usual.

If you've any doubts, talk to your health visitor.

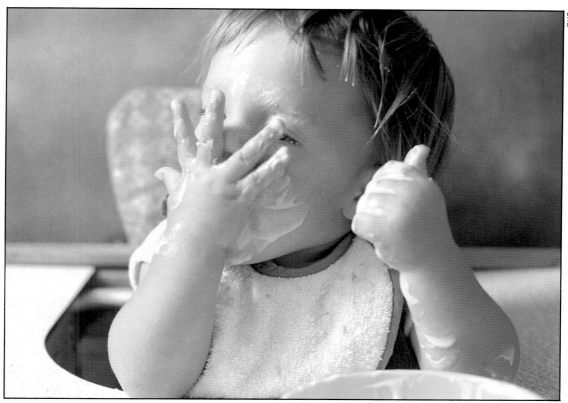

Guidelines

○ It helps to remember the obvious fact that all babies are different. Some start solid food earlier, some later. Some take to it quickly, some take longer. Some are choosy, others like anything and everything.

○ Until now your baby has only known food that is liquid and comes from a nipple or teat. What you are doing is teaching your baby to take and enjoy food that has a different taste, a different feel, and comes in a different way. This is bound to take time. Go at your baby's pace.

○ In the end, you want your baby to be eating like the rest of the family. So your baby needs to learn to like a variety of ordinary foods. In any case, variety early on might mean you avoid choosiness later. Your baby also needs to adapt to the family pattern of eating (say, three meals a day with a drink at each). This too is going to take time.

○ From the start, try not to rush and don't 'force feed'. Most babies know when they've had enough to eat. Don't spend a lot of time persuading your baby to take food. Babies soon learn that refusing food is a good way of getting attention – or of getting a sugary pudding instead of a savoury first course. Of course it's right to give attention, chat, and enjoy meals together. But when food is refused, it might be best to call an end to the meal.

○ Once your baby starts to try and feed him or herself, get ready for the mess and give one spoon to your baby while you spoon in most of the meal. Newspaper on the floor makes cleaning up easier. Babies do find their mouths – sooner or later.

○ When preparing food for your baby, cleanliness is important. Equipment should be really clean. Food standing at room temperature, before or after puréeing, can be a breeding ground for germs. And it's not a good idea to store half-eaten foods.

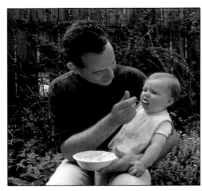

Starting solid food

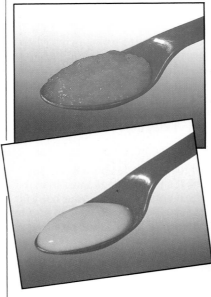

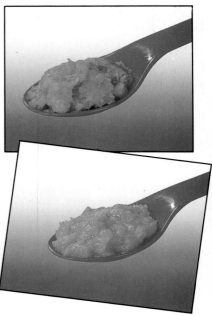

Step 1

Start with a little vegetable or fruit purée (with no added salt or sugar) or cereal (not wheat-based) on the tip of a clean teaspoon or your finger. Just a small teaspoonful is enough at first. Offer it after one milk feed in the day, or in the middle of the feed if that works better for your baby. If you heat the food, make sure it's not too hot when you give it. It's better not to use a microwave oven for this.

Most babies take time to learn how to take food from a spoon. Be patient and prepared for some spitting and mess. Your baby may also cry between mouthfuls at first. Until now, food has come in one continuous stream. Now there are frustrating pauses.

Don't press the food on your baby. If it really doesn't seem to be wanted, give up. Leave it a day, or maybe a week, and then try again.

Once your baby has got the hang of taking solid food from a spoon, say after a week or two, you can move on to Step 2.

Foods you might try: vegetable or fruit purées (potato, carrot, yam, plantain, spinach, apple, banana, etc); thin porridge (made from rice, cornmeal, sago, millet, for example). You can also buy baby rice and other first baby foods in the shops. Use the instructions on the packet to make these up.

Don't yet give: wheat-based foods such as wheat cereals; milk other than breast or formula milk; eggs; citrus fruits; nuts; fatty foods; chillies.

Step 2

Still start feeds with breast or bottle, but now very gradually increase the amount of solid food you give afterwards. Try to follow your baby's appetite. Give the amount that seems to be wanted and no more.

At the same time, move gradually from solid food at one feed in the day to solid food at two, and then three. Again, try to follow your baby's appetite and to go at your baby's pace.

Try to keep cereals for one feed only. Begin to add different foods and different tastes, but take it slowly. Two or three new foods each week is probably fast enough. You'll be able to use lots of the foods you already cook for yourself. Just mash, sieve or purée a small amount (without added salt or sugar) and give it a try. Using your own family food is cheaper, but you know what the ingredients are (halal meat, for example), and your baby will get used to eating like the rest of the family more quickly.

Foods you might now add: purées using meat (including liver), poultry, fish, and split pulses such as lentils; a wider variety of vegetable and fruit purées.

Still avoid: wheat-based foods; milk other than breast or formula milk; eggs; citrus fruits; nuts; fatty foods; chillies.

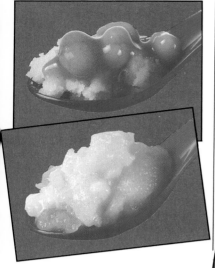

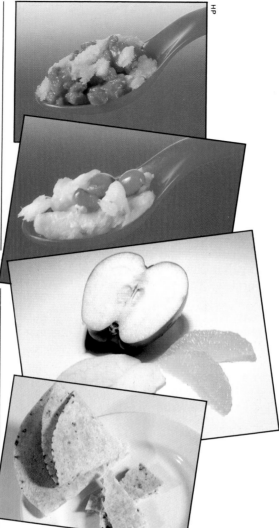

Step 3

Once your baby has grown used to a variety of foods, you can begin to give the solids first and the milk feed second.

It is a good idea to carry on with breast or bottle in the first year. You can begin to use cow's milk after six months for mixing food; and as a drink after the first year. Use whole pasteurised milk. Semi-skimmed, skimmed or unpasteurised milk (usually with a green top) shouldn't be given to young children. You can also move on to the odd drink of diluted natural fruit juice or water as a drink with meals.

Foods you could now add:
wheat-based foods; dairy foods (yogurt and cottage cheese, for example); citrus fruits; smooth peanut butter. In other words, you can now give almost any family food, provided you can make it the right consistency for your baby.

(For information about healthy eating for the whole family, see pages 46-49.)

Step 4

Your baby will gradually learn to cope with food that's lumpier. You can move on from purées to food that's just mashed with a fork or minced.

Once your baby can hold and handle things, try giving a piece of peeled apple, a scrubbed carrot, a crust of bread, or a bit of pitta bread or chappatti. This gives good chewing practice and it will help your baby to learn to feed himself or herself. Stay nearby, in case of choking. Avoid things like sweet biscuits and rusks, so your baby doesn't get into the habit of expecting sweet snacks. Even low-sugar rusks contain sugar.

When your baby begins to chew, you will only have to chop up food. And pieces of fruit, sandwiches, toast etc can become part of a day's menu.

FOODS TO WATCH

Salt Don't add salt to your baby's food. A small baby's system can't cope with more salt than is naturally found in foods. When you're cooking for the family, leave out the salt so your baby can share the food. Cutting down on salt is generally good for everyone – see page 49.

Sugar Adding extra sugar to your baby's food or drinks can give a taste for sweet things which can lead to tooth decay problems later. Try to give savoury foods as much as possible. If you use tins or packets of baby food, look for the ones without added sugar. There are now some on the market. Read the labels: watch out for glucose, sucrose, dextrose, fructose, maltose, syrup, honey, raw/brown sugar or concentrated fruit juice.
Watch out for foods and drinks which claim to be low in sugar but actually contain quite a lot.

Wheat cereals, eggs and **citrus fruits** sometimes cause allergic reactions. Wait until your baby is about six months old before you start giving them. Then introduce them in small quantities and one at a time, so you can watch for any reaction. (Egg yolk is more digestible than egg white, so start with the yolk only.) If anyone in your immediate family suffers from allergies, it's possible your baby might too, so talk to your doctor or health visitor first.

Eggs should be thoroughly cooked until the white and yolk are solid.

Cow's, goat's, and **sheep's milk** may cause allergic reactions. Goat's milk is also low in folic acid, one of the important vitamins. If you do use goat's or sheep's milks, you will need to boil them first then let them cool, because the law doesn't require that they are pasteurised.

Nuts shouldn't be given to babies and small children because of the risk of choking. Finely ground nuts may be given after six months.

Weaning from the breast or bottle

You can go on breast feeding your baby, alongside giving solid food, for as long as you want to. If both you and your baby enjoy it, there's no reason to stop. A bedtime breast feed can make a good end to the day.

Continuing breast feeding or using infant formula during the first year ensures a good source of nutrients as well as being convenient and cheap.

Weaning from the bottle is more important. Comfort sucking on a bottle or dinky feeder can become a habit that's hard to break. And if the drink is sweet, it can cause very bad tooth decay. Try to wean your baby off the bottle (or a dinky feeder) by the age of one.

Start with a lidded feeding cup. Offer the breast or bottle as well at first, and gradually cut down. Or, if you think this puts your baby off the cup because there's something 'better' coming afterwards, try cutting out the breast or bottle feed at one meal in the day and using the cup instead. Go on from there.

Crying

"At first, it really upset me. I felt I ought to be able to comfort him, I ought to be able to make him happy, and he *wasn't* happy, and I *couldn't* comfort him, no matter what I did. And then it went on so long, it felt like forever, and I was still upset but I got sort of worn out by it, almost angry, because I was so disappointed that things weren't like I wanted them to be. I wanted to enjoy him, and I wanted him to be like other babies, smiling, gurgling, all of that, and he was just dreadful with the crying."

"It was every evening, we'd be there, rocking her and walking up and down. We got so exhausted we were desperate. And then it stopped, gradually. It's like everything like that goes on for at least a month longer than you think you can bear, but you do bear it, because there's nothing else for it. And in the end, it stops."

A lot of people seem to think that babies shouldn't cry. They think that if babies *do* cry, there must be a reason and you, the parent, should be able to do something about it.

But all babies cry, and some cry a lot. Sometimes you will know the reason. If your baby is crying from hunger, or a dirty nappy, tiredness, or even loneliness or boredom, then you will know what to do about it. But often you won't know the reason, all you can do is try to find ways of comforting your baby.

Try:

○ letting your baby suckle at the breast.

○ holding your baby close, rocking, swaying, talking, singing.

○ rocking backwards and forwards in the pram, or going out for a walk or a drive. Quite a lot of babies sleep in cars and even if your baby wakes up again the minute you stop, you've at least had a break.

○ putting your baby in a sling, held close against you. Move gently about, sway, dance.

○ things to look at or listen to. Music on the radio or tape, a rattle, a mobile above the cot.

○ a dummy, sterilised for small babies, never sweetened. Some babies find their thumb instead. Others will use a muslin or some other bit of cloth as a comforter and you can wash this as often as you need.

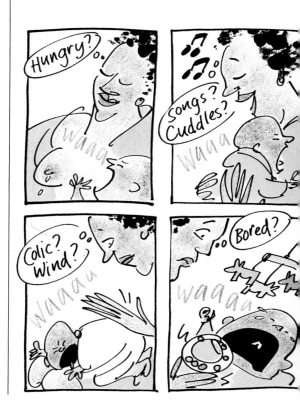

○ firm, rhythmic stroking, with your baby held against you or lying face downwards on your lap. Or undress your baby and massage with baby oil, gently and firmly. Talk soothingly as you do it. Make sure the room is warm enough.

○ a warm bath. This calms some babies instantly – but makes others cry even more. Like everything else, it might be worth a try.

○ Some babies seem to reach a point when they just don't want to be handled any more. You might try making your baby comfortable in the cot or pram and letting him or her be for a little while. See what happens.

Colic

Many babies have particular times in the day when they cry and cry and are difficult to comfort. The early evening is the usual bad patch. This is hard on you since it's probably the time when you are most tired and least able to cope.

Crying like this can be due to colic. Everybody agrees that colic exists, but there is disagreement about what it really is. Some doctors say that it is a kind of stomach cramp, and it does seem to cause the kind of crying that might go with waves of stomach pain – very miserable and distressed, stopping for a moment or two, then starting up again. The crying can go on for some hours, and there may be little you can do except try to comfort your baby, and wait for the crying to pass.

○ Try holding your baby in a way that puts gentle pressure and warmth on his or her stomach. Say, face down across your lap, or against your shoulder. Rhythmically rub and stroke your baby's back.

○ If you are breast feeding, it may be that something in *your* diet is upsetting your baby. When your baby seems colicky and uncomfortable, it may be worth looking back over what you've eaten in the last 24 hours. If there's something you think might be the cause of the problem, you could try cutting it out for a while.

○ A drug which was given for colic in the past has been taken off the market as unsafe. But there are now some new medicines which are safe for babies and may help. If colic is a real problem, see your doctor.

A lot of babies go through a colicky phase and it can last for some weeks. The phase does pass eventually. Try to hold onto this. In the meantime, organise life so you are better able to cope. If you know that your baby will be in your arms all evening, needing all your attention and energy, eat a good meal at lunchtime and try to get a sleep in the afternoon. Share comforting with your partner, or someone else, to spread the strain.

If the strain gets too much

Comforting a crying baby can be exhausting and stressful. When you're tired anyway, when you've tried everything and nothing seems to work, it's normal to feel desperate, angry, and as though you can't take any more. Think about:

○ handing your baby over to someone else for an hour. Nobody can cope alone with a constantly crying baby. You need someone who will give you a break, at least every now and then, to calm down and get some rest.

○ putting your baby down in the cot or pram and going away for a while. Make sure your baby's safe, close the door, go into another room or walk outside, and do what you can to calm yourself down. Set a time limit – say, ten minutes – and then go back.

○ Ask your health visitor if she knows of any local support for parents of crying babies. Some areas run a telephone helpline. An organisation called Cry-sis has branches in many areas and offers support through mothers who have had crying babies themselves. See page 94 for details of this and other support organisations.

> Crying is sometimes a sign of illness. If you are worried for any reason, if the crying seems different from usual, or if there's anything else unusual about the way your baby looks or behaves, then contact your doctor. See page 21 for what do to if you think your baby may be ill.

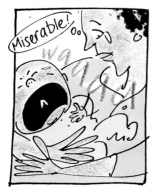
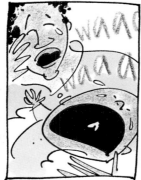

Sleeping

"A friend of mine had a baby about the same time as me and he was one of those babies who's always slept, you know, so you could almost set your watch by him. I'd go round to see her, and I'd have been up most of the night with Paul, and say, he might have had the odd hour in the morning, and she'd be there, with the baby asleep, getting on with her jobs, and she'd not have been up once in the night."

Some babies sleep much more than others. Some sleep in long patches, some in short. Some sleep through the night early, some not for a long time. Your baby will develop his or her own pattern of waking and sleeping, and it is unlikely to be the same as other babies you know. Also, the pattern will change over time.

One thing is certain. Your baby's sleeping pattern is very unlikely to fit in with *your* need for sleep.

At the start, try to follow your baby's needs. You'll gradually get to know when sleep is needed. Snatch sleep and rest for yourself whenever you can.

A baby who wants to sleep isn't likely to be disturbed by household noise. So there's no need to keep the house silent while your baby sleeps. It will help you if your child gets used to sleeping through a certain amount of noise.

You shouldn't leave your baby alone with a bottle as a way of getting off to sleep. There's a danger of choking.

A baby who always falls asleep in a parent's arms, at the breast, or with someone by the cot, may not easily take to settling alone. This may not matter to you. But some parents want their babies to learn to go off to sleep alone.

Later, around three or four months, you may be able to encourage your baby to sleep more at the times you want – such as through the night. Try:

○ waking your baby for a feed just before you go to bed.

○ cutting down a bit on daytime sleeping.

○ making it clear that days are different from nights. Start a bedtime routine, perhaps playing in the bath and then having a quiet time, talking, cuddling, singing or, when your baby is old enough to enjoy it, looking at a picture book. Then, if you're needed in the night, keep lights low and noises soft.

Disturbed nights, week after week, month after month, can be very hard to bear. Share getting up in the night with your partner if you can. If you can't you might be able to go to stay with grandparents or friends who will help you out and give you one or two nights of undisturbed sleep.

See page 43 for more information about sleeping problems in older babies and children.

Cry-sis, the organisation for parents of crying babies (address on page 94), can also offer help with sleeping problems.

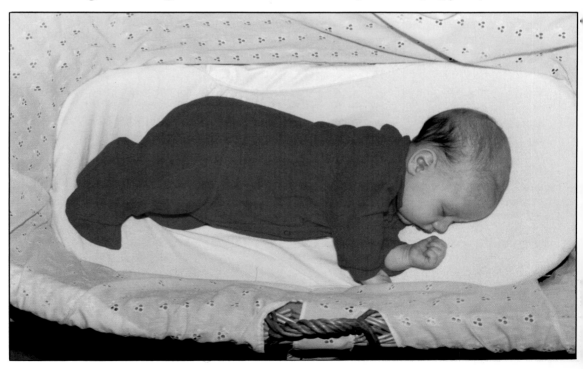

Cot deaths

Reducing the risk

Sadly, we don't yet know why some babies die suddenly and for no apparent reason from what is called cot death or sudden infant death syndrome (SIDS). But we do know that there are ways of reducing the risks.

Sleeping position

Babies laid to sleep on their tummies are more at risk of cot death than babies laid down on their back or side. **So lay your baby to sleep on his or her back or side.**

If you lay your baby on the side, put the lower arm well in front of the body so that your baby doesn't roll forward on to his or her tummy. Don't put wedges or rolled up sheets behind your sleeping baby.

Only lay your baby down to sleep on his or her front if your doctor advises it – this will only be for a particular medical reason.

Temperature

Small babies are not very good at controlling their own temperature. They can't move around to get warm, or kick off the covers if they're too hot, so you need to be careful to keep them at an even temperature.

Indoors

Healthy babies need to be able to lose heat from their head and face, so don't cover them.

Some other important points:
- The rooms in which babies sleep should be neither too hot nor too cold – about 16 – 20°C. As a guide, this should feel comfortable for lightly clothed adults. A thermometer in the room will help to make sure.
- If your home is warm, your baby doesn't need to be wrapped up. An over-dressed baby in a warm room can become dangerously overheated.
- Keep the bedding consistent with the temperature of the room. Again, as a guide, babies need little more bedding than adults.
- Make sure the baby can't slip under the bedding. To avoid this, you can make the bed up so that the baby's feet come down to the end of the cot.
- Duvets should not be used before your baby is a year old.
- Babies should not be exposed to direct heat while they're asleep, for example from a hot water bottle or an electric blanket.
- Babies of one month and over don't need to wear hats indoors for sleeping unless it's very cold.
- Ill or feverish babies do *not* need any extra bedding. In fact, they may well need *less* to cool them down.
- It's fine to take your baby into your bed for a cuddle or a feed. It's not a good idea for the baby to sleep in the bed with you all night because he or she could become overheated or slip beneath the bedclothes.

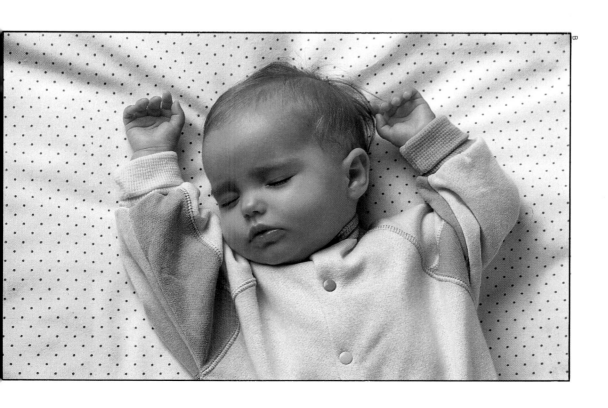

Outdoors

Babies, especially very young babies, can lose heat and chill very quickly when they're taken outdoors in cold weather, so make sure they're well wrapped up. Remember to take off their outdoor clothes – especially hats – when you bring them indoors again, unless it happens to be cold indoors as well. It's all the more important to do this if they're asleep when they're brought indoors – even though there's a risk that you might wake them up!

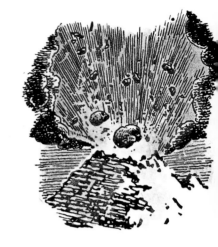

Smoking

Babies should not be exposed to tobacco smoke, either before birth or afterwards. If you, or anyone else who looks after your baby smokes, try not to smoke anywhere near the baby. It would be even better if everyone could make an effort to give up completely. Babies and young children who breathe in cigarette smoke are also more likely to get coughs and chest infections.

Breast feeding

There are many benefits to breast feeding but there is no clear evidence that it reduces the risk of cot death.

If your baby seems at all unwell, seek medical advice early and quickly.

Do remember that cot death is rare. Don't let worrying about cot death spoil the first precious months you have with your baby.

What's in a nappy

Babies' stools can be very brightly coloured, greenish at first, then probably yellow or orange, or greyish green if your baby is bottle fed. Breast-fed babies have quite runny stools. Bottle-fed babies' stools are firmer and smellier.

From day to day or week to week, your baby's stools will probably vary a bit. But if you notice a marked change of any kind, such as the stools becoming very smelly or very watery, contact your doctor or health visitor.

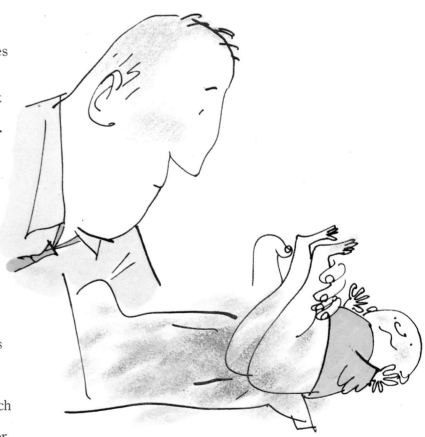

Some babies fill their nappies at or around every feed. Some (especially breast-fed babies), can go for several days, even a week, without a bowel movement. Either is normal. Quite a lot of babies also strain or even cry when passing a stool. This too is normal. It doesn't mean they are constipated so long as the stools are soft. If you do become worried that your baby may be constipated, mention it to your doctor or health visitor.

Nappy rash   Most babies get nappy rash at some time. There may be a rash, or just general soreness. Take extra care over cleaning your baby, with water not soap. Dry well before putting on a clean nappy. Change nappies more often. You may want to use a protective cream, although some parents find it better to let the skin breathe. Air will do the skin good, so it helps to let your baby lie on the changing mat without a nappy for a while. Have a spare nappy or cloth ready to mop up.

If the rash gets very bad or won't go away, ask your health visitor or doctor about it. It may be that your baby has **thrush**, an infection which needs treatment. Your doctor can prescribe a cream which will clear up the infection quite quickly.

In hot weather, protect your baby from the sun with a shade and a sun hat. Babies' skins burn easily, even in sun which wouldn't affect your own skin. In hot sun, use a sun screen cream/lotion.

When you're worried

There are bound to be times when your baby worries you. If you are anxious about something, no matter how small, look for help. The kind of help you need will depend on the worry. In Chapter 6 you will find information about the different kinds of help and support that are available.

The biggest worry of all is that your baby might be ill. It can be difficult to decide whether a baby is ill or not, and difficult to decide whether to see the doctor. Trust your feelings. You know better than anyone what is unusual for your baby. Even if it turns out that nothing is wrong, that is exactly what you need to know.

Some doctors are very supportive towards parents of small babies. Many will fit babies into surgeries without an appointment, or see them at the beginning of surgery hours. Many will give advice over the phone. Others are less helpful. And it's not always easy to phone or to get to the surgery. Even so, if you are worried about a particular problem that won't go away, it's right to persist.

ALWAYS CONTACT YOUR DOCTOR:

– if you think your baby is ill, even if you can't make out what's wrong,
or
– if your baby has one or more of these problems:

Always urgent:

○ a fit (convulsion), or your baby turns blue or very pale

○ quick, difficult or grunting breathing

○ your baby is unusually drowsy or hard to wake, or doesn't seem to know you.

Sometimes serious:

○ a hoarse cough with noisy breathing

○ your baby cries for an unusually long time or in an unusual way or seems to be in a lot of pain

○ your baby keeps refusing feeds

○ diarrhoea or vomiting

○ unusually hot or cold or floppy.

If you have seen your doctor or health visitor and your baby is not getting better or is getting worse, tell your doctor again the same day. If you become worried and you can't get hold of your doctor or your doctor can't come to you quickly enough, then take your baby straight to the accident and emergency department of the nearest hospital with a children's unit. It's worth finding out in advance where this is, in case you ever need it.
(For more information about illness, see pages 52-58.)

"He doesn't seem to listen. I'm in and out in no time, and I come away no better off than if I'd stayed at home. In fact, sometimes it makes it worse, because he'll give me something and I'll not know whether it's really needed or not."

"My doctor gives me advice. He's also a Moslem, you see, so he can give me advice about any questions I want to ask. He said if I had any worries, I could always go and talk to him."

"She always makes me feel that what I've got to say and what I think is important. It gives me a lot of confidence."

When a baby dies

"There was this huge emptiness, and the only way we could fill the emptiness and begin to understand was to talk and talk, and to cry. The real friends were the ones who let us talk and weren't afraid to see us cry. The last thing we wanted was to be helped to feel better. That would have meant forgetting what had happened to us before we'd even begun to live with it. It would have meant forgetting our baby. You never forget. It will always be a part of us. The baby's a part of us, just like any child."

There's a feeling that babies are not *meant* to die. That feeling adds great shock (as well as maybe anger, bewilderment, even a kind of guilt) to the enormous grief and sadness brought by a baby's death. The grief, sadness and other feelings are important to you. They are not to be set aside quickly or hidden away.

You need to let yourself grieve in your own way. If you need to cry, don't hold back the tears. Crying may be the only way of letting out your feelings. If you feel angry, as many parents do, or find you're blaming yourself or others, it's important to talk about it. Ask the questions you want to ask of, for example, hospital staff, your doctor, midwife or health visitor. Often the reasons for a baby's death are never known, not even after a post-mortem. But you need to find out all you can.

After the first shock, it may help you to think about ways of remembering your baby and making him or her remembered. Give a lot of thought to any service or ceremony you may want, and to mementoes you may want to keep.

Try to explain what has happened, as simply and honestly as you can, to any older children. They need to understand why you are sad, and will have their own feelings to cope with. Sometimes an older child connects the death with something he or she has done, and may be very quiet, or badly behaved, for a time. It's not easy for you to give the love and reassurance that's needed. It may help to get support from others close to your child.

Coping with the outside world and other people is difficult at first. You may find that even people quite close to you don't know what to say, say the wrong thing, or avoid you. Take the support that's given and feels right.

It's best to expect a long time of difficult feelings and ups and downs. Talking may not come easily to you, but even some time after your baby's death, it can help to talk about your feelings. The more you and your partner can talk to each other, the more it will help you both. A father's experience of a baby's death can be different from a mother's. Although you will share a lot, your feelings and moods won't be the same all the time. Try to listen to each other so you can support each other as best you can.

Sometimes talking to someone outside the family is helpful – a close friend, your doctor, health visitor, hospital staff, maybe a priest or other religious counsellor. Talking to other parents who have been through the same loss and grief can be a special help. You can contact other parents through these organisations:

The Stillbirth and Neonatal Death Society is run by and for parents whose baby has died either at birth or shortly afterwards.

The Foundation for the Study of Infant Deaths supports parents bereaved by a cot death or what is called 'sudden infant death'.

The Compassionate Friends is an organisation of and for all bereaved parents.

Addresses and phone numbers are on page 95.

"Time goes by and gradually, if you grieve enough, you begin to accept it. A time comes when you can make it all right with yourself to feel happy about happy things."

2. Growing and learning

Growth
Weight/height checks

Checking growth, both in weight and height, is a simple way of checking a child's health and progress.

You can have your baby regularly weighed and measured at your child health clinic or doctor's baby clinic. Older children should be weighed and measured as part of other health checks.

At the clinic, your baby's growth will be recorded on **centile charts**. The lines already printed on the charts show roughly the kind of growth expected, in weight and in length. The middle, heavy line represents the national average.

Of course there is no reason why your baby should be 'average'. In fact, these centile charts were developed some time ago, using a white British population. As a result, the averages shown are not right for some ethnic groups. The average birth weights and heights in some groups is slightly different. Variations between ethnic groups need to be taken into account when using the charts.

It doesn't matter where your baby starts on the chart. Whatever weight and length your baby was at birth, there should be fairly steady growth, with a line curving in *roughly* the same way as the lines on the chart. During the first two years of life, it is quite usual for a baby's line to cross the lines on the chart. But if at anytime your baby's weight line suddenly goes up or drops (and it may drop, for example, because of illness), talk to your health visitor about it. Talk to your health visitor too if, after the age of two, your baby's height line does not follow a centile line or stops altogether.

Babies do vary in how fast they put on weight. What is looked for is not so much a steady week-by-week gain as a general gain over a period of time. For most babies, weight gain is quickest in the first six to nine months, and then slows. As a rough guide, most babies double their birthweight by six months and treble it by a year.

You may have a chart that is slightly different from the one pictured here but it works in the same way.

Boys and girls have different charts because boys are on average heavier and taller and their growth pattern is slightly different.

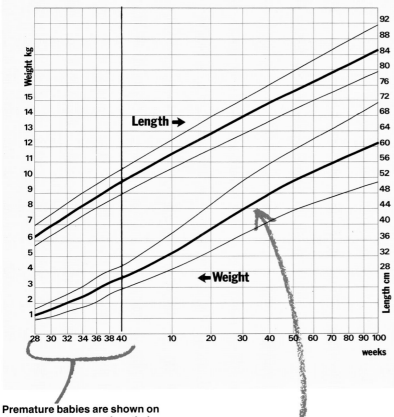

Girls

Premature babies are shown on the chart as younger than their real age. Their starting point on the chart is the week of pregnancy in which they are born. So, for example, a baby born in the 36th week of pregnancy will reach the ten week point on the chart when really 14 weeks old.

The middle line is called the 50th centile, meaning that the weight or length of 50 per cent of children fall on or above the line, and 50 per cent on or below it. The two outer lines are the 3rd and 97th centiles. Only 3 per cent of babies fall outside each of these lines, meaning that they are very small or very big.

Development

(A father) "**When he does something new that he's never done before, that's magic. It's like no other baby in the world has ever done it.**"

"**My mum said, 'Isn't she walking yet?' And as it happened, the little boy next door who's about the same age was up and walking, and Annie was just sitting there not doing a thing. My mum said I was walking at that age. She kept going on about it.**"

(A father) "**I want to know that she's all right, and you know, keeping up**"

Babies and small children grow and develop at such different rates, it's hard to know what is 'normal'. It can be 'normal' for a child to be walking at one, and equally 'normal' for a one year old not even to be crawling, let alone walking. A two and a half year old might be talking very clearly, or might talk a lot but still be hard to understand. Each child is different.

Children develop differently because each is an individual. They also develop differently because their experiences are different. Parents and families vary. There may be two parents or one, there may be one child or more, parents may be in paid work or at home . . . Some children play a lot with toys, some don't; some are taken out and about a lot, others aren't; some have a lot of contact with different adults and other children, others have less . . . And so on. All these things affect a child's development, but there is nothing about any of them that is right or wrong. It's the experience that counts, and making the most of it, whatever it might be.

The more opportunities babies and children have to do things, and the more encouragement they get, the more likely they are to do them. They need to try out new skills. They will take any kind of opportunity you can give them to do that.

For more about play and learning, see pages 31-33.

A Guide to Development

This guide gives an idea of the age range within which *most* children gain certain skills. The ages given are averages. Lots of perfectly normal children gain one skill earlier, another later than average.

See page 29 for what to do if you're worried.

Movement

Most children:

☐ lift their heads by about 3 months.

☐ sit without support between 6 and 8 months. If your baby is not sitting unsupported by 9 months, talk to your health visitor or doctor.

☐ start *trying* to crawl around 6 months. Some crawl backwards before they crawl forwards. Crawling may really get going around 9 months. But some children learn to walk without ever crawling at all. Others are bottom-shufflers.

☐ pull themselves upright and stand, holding onto the furniture, between 6 and 10 months.

☐ walk alone between 10 and 16 months. If your child is not walking by 18 months, talk to your health visitor or doctor.

☐ learn to kick or throw a ball between 18 months and 2 years Throwing sometimes takes longer than kicking.

☐ learn to pedal a trike between about 2 and 3 years.

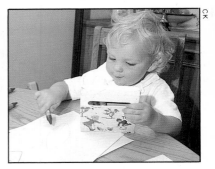

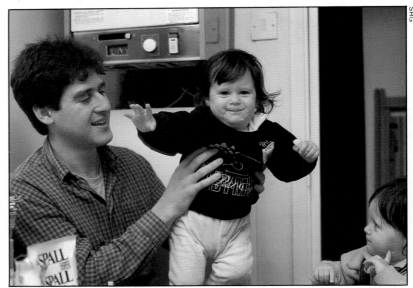

Handling things

Most children:

☐ will reach out for objects between 3 and 5 months.

☐ can hold an object and will lift it up to suck it between 5 and 8 months. At first, babies can hold objects but not let go. At about 6 to 7 months, they learn to pass things from hand to hand, maybe via their mouths. They learn to let go of things (for example, to drop something, or give it to you) at about 9 to 10 months.

☐ use both their right and left hands, without preference, until about 3 years old

☐ can feed themselves the sort of foods they can pick up and hold at about 10 months.

☐ begin to feed themselves, very messily, with a spoon sometime after 14 months.

☐ begin to take off easy clothes (like loose, short socks) from about 14 months.

☐ begin to be able to build bricks between 15 and 18 months. Large bricks are easiest to start with.

☐ enjoy scribbling with a crayon from about 18 months onwards.

☐ can draw what you can see is a person (with a face and maybe arms and legs) between 3 and 4 years old. Like much else, this depends a lot on how much practice and encouragement they get.

Hearing and talking

Babies react to noise from very early on. Watch how your baby responds to sounds. It is often parents themselves who pick up any problems to do with hearing.

The development of talking has a lot to do with how much babies are talked to. Chatting to your baby is important from the start. Later, a child who is talked to a lot will not just copy the words that he or she hears but also invent language and learn to like using it.

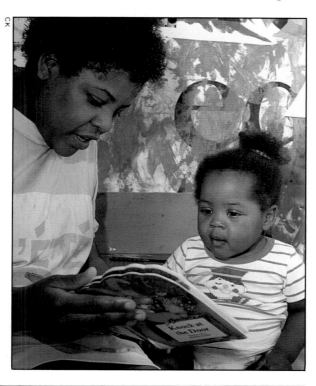

If you are ever worried about your child's language development, talk to your doctor or health visitor. You can ask to be referred to a speech therapist.

Children who are growing up to speak two languages don't usually have problems, and later it is a great advantage. A few develop language a bit more slowly. The important thing is to talk to your child in whatever language you feel most at home with. This may mean one parent mostly using one language, the other parent using another. Children usually adapt to this.

Most children:

☐ are startled by sudden, loud noises from birth.

☐ make cooing noises from about 3 months.

☐ by 3 months will quieten to the sound of a parent's voice, and may turn towards the sound.

☐ by 6 months are making repetitive noises, like 'gagaga . . .' and enjoy making more and more different sounds.

☐ start to use particular sounds for particular things between 10 and 14 months.

☐ say something like 'mama' and 'dada' to anyone from about 6 to 9 months and to their parents from 10 to 12 months.

☐ by 18 months, can say between 6 and 20 recognisable single words, but understand much more than they can say. They also start to use language in play – for example, when feeding a teddy or doll, or talking on a toy telephone.

☐ can put at least two words together by 2 years old, and can point to parts of their body.

☐ can talk well in sentences and chant rhymes and songs by 3 years old.

☐ by 3 years old are talking clearly enough to be understood by strangers. A few 3 year olds may still be difficult to understand. It is normal for a 2 year old to pronounce words wrongly.

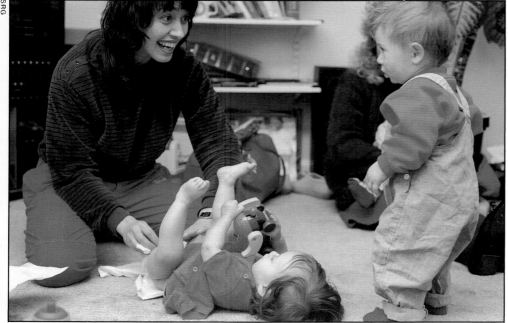

Seeing

Babies can see from birth, but for a few months they can only focus on what is close to them. So to begin with, the other side of a room, for example, is a blur, but a face close in front of them is clear – and interesting. The distance they can see gradually increases.

Many babies squint at birth. If you still notice the squint after three to four months, you should ask your doctor about it.

Most children:

☐ begin to recognise their parents by 2 weeks, and start to smile at around 4 to 6 weeks

☐ in the first few weeks, especially like looking at faces. They will focus on a face close in front of them, and follow it. They prefer the face of a parent, or a known face, to a strange one.

☐ can follow a brightly coloured moving toy, held about 20cm/8ins away, by about 6 weeks.

☐ can see across a room by about 6 months.

For information about development checks for your child, see page 28.

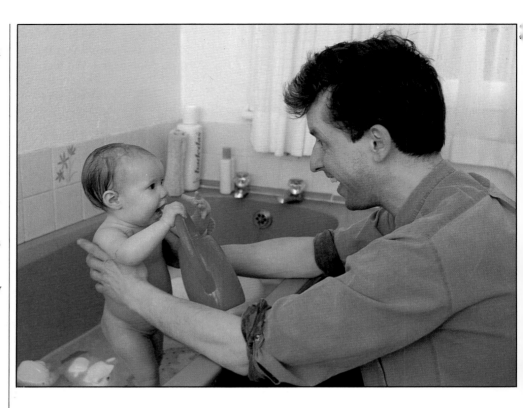

What happens, and when?

This chart will give you some idea of what happens in a child's development. Each band on the chart shows the span of time within which you might expect your child to start doing something.

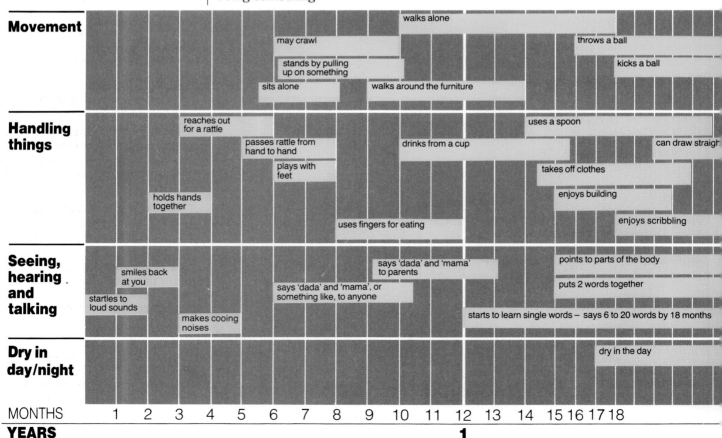

	Movement
	walks alone
	may crawl
	stands by pulling up on something
	sits alone
	walks around the furniture
	throws a ball
	kicks a ball

Handling things
- reaches out for a rattle
- passes rattle from hand to hand
- plays with feet
- holds hands together
- drinks from a cup
- uses fingers for eating
- uses a spoon
- takes off clothes
- enjoys building
- enjoys scribbling
- can draw straight

Seeing, hearing and talking
- startles to loud sounds
- smiles back at you
- makes cooing noises
- says 'dada' and 'mama', or something like, to anyone
- says 'dada' and 'mama' to parents
- starts to learn single words – says 6 to 20 words by 18 months
- points to parts of the body
- puts 2 words together

Dry in day/night
- dry in the day

MONTHS   1 2 3 4 5 6 7 8 9 10 11 12 13 14 15 16 17 18
YEARS   1

26

Teeth

The times when babies get their first teeth (milk teeth) varies. A few are born with a tooth already through. Others have no teeth at one year old. Most get their first tooth at around six months, usually in front, at the bottom. Most have all their primary teeth by about two and a half. The first secondary (permanent) teeth come through at the back around the age of six.

There are 20 primary (first) teeth in all, ten at the top, ten at the bottom.

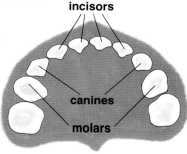

Teething can bring problems, though some teeth seem to come through with no pain or trouble at all. You may notice the gum is sore and red where the tooth is coming, or that one cheek is flushed. Your baby may dribble, gnaw and chew

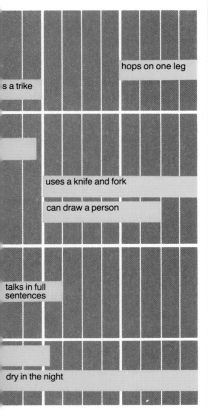

a lot, or just be fretful, but it's often hard to tell whether this is really due to teething.

It can help to give your baby something hard to chew on – a teething ring, a dried crust of bread, a scrubbed carrot (stay nearby in case of choking). Avoid rusks because almost all contain some sugar. Constant chewing and sucking on sugary things can cause bad tooth decay, even when there are only one or two teeth. If you think a tooth is really hurting, teething gel rubbed on the gum, or one 5ml spoon of baby paracetamol, might help. You can get these from the chemist. It's possible to get sugar-free teething gel.

People put all sorts of things down to teething – rashes, crying, bad temper, runny noses, extra dirty nappies. But be careful not to explain away what might be signs of illness by saying it's 'just teething'.

(See page 50 for information about how to care for your child's teeth.)

Feet - and first shoes

Babies' and small children's feet grow very fast and it's important that the bones grow straight.

○ A baby's toes are curly at birth. If they are cramped by tight bootees, socks, stretch suits or pram shoes, the toes can't straighten out. So keep your baby's feet as free as possible. Make sure bootees, socks etc. leave room for the toes, both in length and width. If the feet of a stretch suit become too small, cut them off, hem the edges, and use socks instead.

○ Don't put your child into proper shoes until he or she can walk alone.

○ When you buy shoes, it's best to have them fitted. They should be fitted about 2cm (¾in) beyond the longest toe and wide enough for all the toes to lie flat.

'Multi-fit' shoes, which you buy in chain stores or mail order, are cheaper but only come in one width fitting. They only fit about half of all British children – those who are D or E fitting. If you buy these shoes, or get shoes secondhand, check fit carefully. Make sure there's plenty of room for the toes,

and also that the shoe isn't too loose. Don't use secondhand shoes which have misshapen soles.

○ Shoes with a lace, buckle or velcro fastening hold the heel in place and stop the foot slipping forward, damaging the toes. If the heel of a shoe slips off when your child stands on tiptoe, it doesn't fit.

○ Leather shoes mould to the shape of the feet, absorb sweat, and let feet breathe. But leather is expensive. If you can't afford it, buy something cheap and throw the shoes away as soon as they're worn out. Have your child's feet measured again for a new pair.

○ Check that socks are the right size.

○ If you have any worry to do with your child's feet, see your doctor or health visitor. You may be able to get free chiropody for your child at your local health clinic. If not, you should go to a state registered chiropodist.

How to check the length of a child's shoes

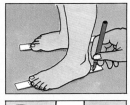

1. Cut two thin strips of cardboard. Get your child to stand on them in bare feet.

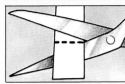

2. Mark the longest toe and the back of the heel.

3. Cut at the marks. Slip the strips into the shoes so that one end touches the toe of the shoe.

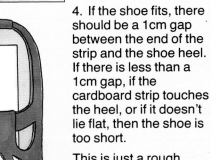

4. If the shoe fits, there should be a 1cm gap between the end of the strip and the shoe heel. If there is less than a 1cm gap, if the cardboard strip touches the heel, or if it doesn't lie flat, then the shoe is too short.

This is just a rough guide. If you can, have shoes fitted or checked by a trained shoe fitter.

Learning to use a potty

Different children gain bladder and bowel control at different ages; it's best not to compare your child with others. Most children can control their bowels before their bladders.

Only one in two children are dry during the day by the age of two. But by the age of three, nine out of ten are dry most days. Even then, *all* children have the odd accident, especially when they're excited, or upset, or absorbed in doing something.

It usually takes longer for a child to be dry at night. At the age of three, two thirds of all children are dry most nights. That means it's not unusual for a three year old to be in nappies at night. Most but by no means all children are dry at night by the age of five.

"It's hard not to push them. You see these other children, you know, younger than yours, and they're all using the potty or the toilet, and there's yours, still in nappies . . . But they all learn in the end, and looking back, it wasn't that important. At the time, I thought it was dreadful because Al was the only child at his playgroup in nappies. But it was only me that minded. Al certainly didn't care, so what does it matter?"

"My mother-in-law kept telling me that all her three were potty trained by a year. At the time, I didn't know whether to believe her or not. I mean, it didn't really seem possible, but I wasn't sure. Looking back now, I suppose she must have spent a lot of time just putting her children on the potty. They didn't really know what they were doing, but if there was something in the potty, she counted that as potty trained. Well, for a start, I haven't got the time or patience for that. And anyway, it doesn't seem worth it. Just catching what comes isn't the same as potty training."

Starting potty training   Some parents start teaching their child to use a potty very early; some don't bother about it until their child actually *asks* to come out of nappies. Many parents seem to think about starting around 18-24 months – but there's no particular time when success is guaranteed. It's probably easier to start in the summer, when washing dries better and there are fewer clothes, if any, to take off.

Try to work out when your child is ready. Most children go through three stages in developing bladder control:

1.   They become aware of having a wet or dirty nappy.

2.   They get to know when they are passing urine (and may tell you they're doing it!)

3.   They know when they *need* to pass urine (and may say so in advance).

You'll probably do best if your child is at stage 3 before you start potty training.

Teaching your child to use the potty is much the same as teaching other things. See page 34 for some suggestions. For coping with problems, see page 44.

Development checks

Development checks are usually offered at these ages:

6–8 weeks
7–9 months
12–18 months
2½–3½ years
Just before or just after starting school.

Timing varies a bit from place to place. Your health visitor will tell you when there are checks for your child. If you are concerned about something at any other time, don't wait for a check. Ask to see someone.

Developmental checks are usually carried out by your health visitor in agreement with your family doctor or clinic doctor. The aim is to spot any problems as early as possible, so it's worth having the checks even if you think your child is doing fine. The checks also give you a chance to talk and ask any questions you want to about your child's health, development or general behaviour.

Each development check will include a general check of your child's health, and development tests suited to your child's age. (Speech and language checks are included.) So, in later checks for example, your child may be asked to do things like building bricks, looking at and talking about pictures, and so on. By watching your child do these things, and by talking with you, the doctor or health visitor can get some idea of your child's abilities and progress.

Many children won't do things at a check-up that they do easily at home. If this happens, tell the doctor or health visitor. Also say if your child is being asked to do something that he or she isn't used to doing. Some skills are assessed through particular sorts of play, such as drawing. A child who doesn't do much drawing or colouring at home may find this hard and it's best to explain why.

Don't, in any case, think of the check as a test that your child either passes or fails. It's not unusual for a child to be slower in one area of development, nor need this be a sign of a problem. But it is a reason for keeping an eye on progress.

If your child's first language isn't English, you may need to ask for development checks to be carried out by someone who can speak your child's language. See page 86 for information about linkworkers.

Hearing and eyesight checks

Your child's eyesight and hearing will also be tested, either as part of a development check or separately. In most areas, hearing is tested at around 7 to 8 months, but if you are worried about your child's hearing or eyesight before this or at any time, ask for an appointment at your clinic or with your family doctor. It is often parents who are the first to suspect a problem. And the earlier a problem is found, the earlier it can be treated.

Hearing tests are very simple but do pick up problems. A hearing problem can affect a child's whole development, so it's very important to find out about it as soon as possible. Still, it's worth remembering that it's quite common for babies not to respond to a hearing test the first time and to need a second test. Also, a large number of children have hearing problems which are just temporary.

Is everything all right?

"When she does something for the first time, it's like it's my achievement as well as hers. I feel proud of her, but I'm proud of myself, too. And then when something doesn't happen, or there's a problem, I feel that's down to me as well. I need somebody to be able to say to me sometimes, 'She's fine. You're doing a good job. There's nothing to worry about'. Or else I need them to tell me what I *could* do to help, or how long I ought to wait, or give me an explanation, so I know it's not all me."

Nobody knows your child like you do. Only parents know how their children behave day to day, know their characters, their likes and dislikes, their difficulties and achievements. Doctors, health visitors and other professionals caring for children don't have this kind of knowledge. But they do know about, and have a lot of experience of, children *generally*. And they offer medical or other expertise as well.

So, if you are worried about your child's development, or about anything else, go to your doctor, health visitor or clinic. Go more than once if you have to. Explain your worry,

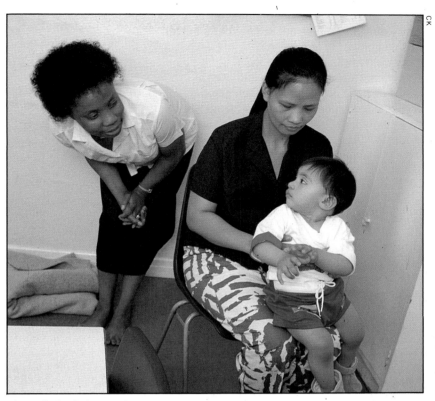

give all the information you can, and ask all the questions you want to ask. If you can put what *you* know together with what the *professionals* know, you stand a better chance of finding the advice or information you need.

Getting to a surgery or clinic is not always easy, especially with a small child or children with you. Not all professionals give you as much time or listen to you as carefully as you want them to. So you may need to be determined. See page 86 for more information about using the services.

Children with special needs

For some families, everything is not 'all right'. Sometimes what begins as a worry does turn out to be a long-term problem or handicap.

If this happens to you, your first need will be for information about the problem and what it is likely to mean for your child and for you. You will have a lot of questions. Put them all to your doctor, your health visitor, and to specialists to whom you are referred. Be determined and persist if you need to. Not all doctors talk easily or well to parents. And you yourself may find it's difficult to hear and take in all that is said to you, first or even second time round. Rather than live with unanswered questions, go back and ask again for the information or opinion you feel you need. If in the end the honest answer is 'I don't know' or 'We're not sure', that's better than no answer at all.

In some areas, there are 'child development teams' or 'district handicap teams'. These are teams of professionals (doctors, therapists, health visitors, social workers) who support children with special needs and their families. You can be referred to such a team through your doctor or health visitor.

You can also get information, advice and support from voluntary organisations. There are a great number of organisations dealing with particular handicaps, illnesses and other problems. Through them, you can often contact other parents in situations like your own. See page 95 for the names and addresses of some organisations to contact.

There are many services available to help children who have special needs to learn and develop: for example, physiotherapy, speech therapy, occupational therapy, home learning schemes, play groups, opportunity groups, nurseries, and nursery schools and classes. To find out what is available in your area, ask your health visitor, social services department, or the educational adviser for special needs at your local education department. (See pages 83-84 for more information about the services – including information about regional variations.)

Local education authorities who think a child over two years old may have special needs must make an assessment of his or her needs. For a child under two, an assessment must be made if a parent asks for it. This assessment is a way of getting advice about your child's educational needs. You can take part in the assessment yourself. The Advisory Centre for Education (address on page 94) offers advice on education and produces a handbook, 'Under-5's with special needs'.

At whatever stage in your child's life you receive a diagnosis of handicap or illness, you will have difficult feelings to cope with, and some hard decisions and adjustments to make. Your doctor, health visitor, social worker, or counsellors of various kinds may all be able to help. So may other parents who have been through similar experiences. But even with help, all parents say it takes time. Throughout that time and afterwards, it is right to think about your own life and needs as well as about your child's.

For information about social security benefits for children with special needs, see page 93. See also 'Help with national health service costs', page 92.

Learning

Play

"I'd play with them all the time if I could. I tell you, it's more fun than doing the housework."

"There are things I've got to do. She's forever asking me to play, and I'm forever saying 'in a minute, in a minute'."

"I don't know that we play all that much. We do a lot of things together, but it's often the shopping, and hanging out the washing, and that sort of thing. It may not be play, but we have a good time."

Children like playing and they need to play. It is through play that they develop new skills and learn about their world, about people and about themselves.

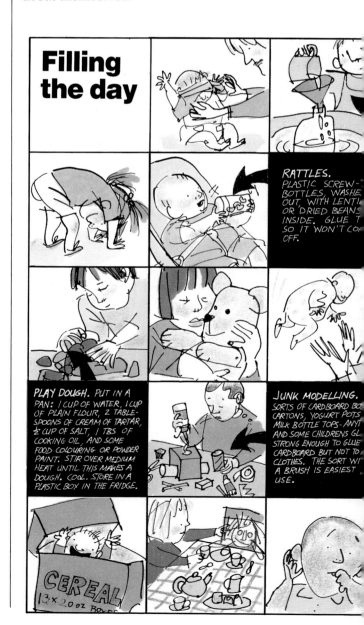

Filling the day

RATTLES. PLASTIC SCREW-TOP BOTTLES, WASHED OUT, WITH LENTILS OR DRIED BEANS INSIDE. GLUE TOP SO IT WON'T COME OFF.

PLAY DOUGH. PUT IN A PAN: 1 CUP OF WATER, 1 CUP OF PLAIN FLOUR, 2 TABLESPOONS OF CREAM OF TARTAR, ½ CUP OF SALT, 1 TBS OF COOKING OIL, AND SOME FOOD COLOURING OR POWDER PAINT. STIR OVER MEDIUM HEAT UNTIL THIS MAKES A DOUGH. COOL. STORE IN A PLASTIC BOX IN THE FRIDGE.

JUNK MODELLING. SORTS OF CARDBOARD BOXES, CARTONS, YOGURT POTS, MILK BOTTLE TOPS- ANYTHING AND SOME CHILDRENS GLUE STRONG ENOUGH TO GLUE CARDBOARD BUT NOT TO CLOTHES. THE SORT WITH A BRUSH IS EASIEST TO USE.

CEREAL 13 x 20 oz Boxes

But young children don't play for long alone. They learn that gradually. In the meantime, play demands your time and attention and you won't be able to give that all the time.

Playing with you is important. But children learn from everything that's going on around them, and everything they do. The times when they are not learning much are the times when they are bored. That's as true of babies as of older children. So what really matters is:

– filling your child's day. That means finding a lot of different things for your child to look at, think about and do. It means making what *you're* doing fun and interesting for your child, so you can get it done; and, sometimes, giving all your attention to what *your child* wants to do.

– finding ways of enjoying each other's company and having fun together, no matter how.

– *talking* about anything and everything, even about the washing up or what to put on the shopping list, so that you share as much as possible.

All of this seems to work best when you're not too organised about it. If you try to work to a strict timetable, your child's very unlikely to fit in with it. Then you both get frustrated. Some things do have to happen at certain times, and your child does slowly have to learn about that. But a lot can be pushed around to suit your mood and your child's. There's no rule that says the washing up has to be done *before* you go to the playground, especially if the sun's shining and your child is bursting with energy.

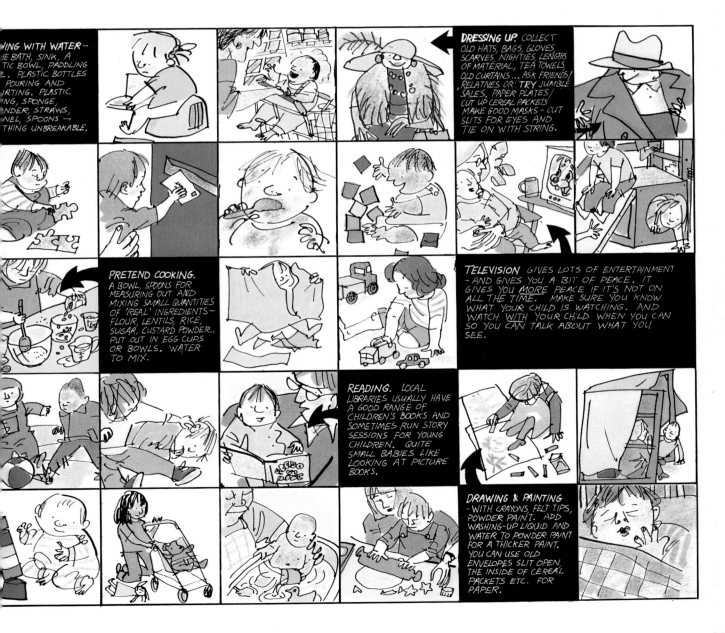

WING WITH WATER – HE BATH, SINK, A TIC BOWL, PADDLING L. PLASTIC BOTTLES POURING AND IRTING. PLASTIC NG, SPONGE, NDER, STRAWS, NEL, SPOONS – THING UNBREAKABLE.

DRESSING UP. COLLECT OLD HATS, BAGS, GLOVES, SCARVES, NIGHTIES, LENGTHS OF MATERIAL, TEA TOWELS, OLD CURTAINS... ASK FRIENDS/ RELATIVES OR TRY JUMBLE SALES. PAPER PLATES/ CUT UP CEREAL PACKETS MAKE GOOD MASKS – CUT SLITS FOR EYES AND TIE ON WITH STRING.

PRETEND COOKING. A BOWL, SPOONS FOR MEASURING OUT AND MIXING SMALL QUANTITIES OF 'REAL' INGREDIENTS– FLOUR, LENTILS, RICE, SUGAR, CUSTARD POWDER.. PUT OUT IN EGG CUPS OR BOWLS. WATER TO MIX.

TELEVISION GIVES LOTS OF ENTERTAINMENT – AND GIVES YOU A BIT OF PEACE. IT GIVES YOU MORE PEACE IF IT'S NOT ON ALL THE TIME. MAKE SURE YOU KNOW WHAT YOUR CHILD IS WATCHING. AND WATCH WITH YOUR CHILD WHEN YOU CAN SO YOU CAN TALK ABOUT WHAT YOU SEE.

READING. LOCAL LIBRARIES USUALLY HAVE A GOOD RANGE OF CHILDREN'S BOOKS AND SOMETIMES RUN STORY SESSIONS FOR YOUNG CHILDREN. QUITE SMALL BABIES LIKE LOOKING AT PICTURE BOOKS.

DRAWING & PAINTING – WITH CRAYONS, FELT TIPS, POWDER PAINT. ADD WASHING-UP LIQUID AND WATER TO POWDER PAINT FOR A THICKER PAINT. YOU CAN USE OLD ENVELOPES SLIT OPEN, THE INSIDE OF CEREAL PACKETS ETC. FOR PAPER.

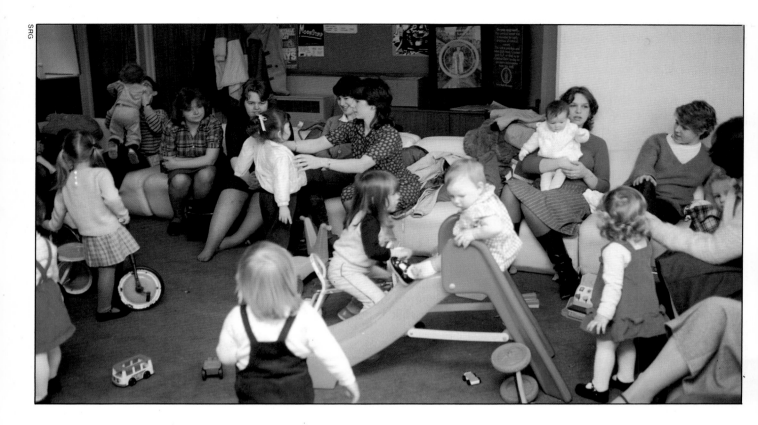

Playing and learning in groups

Children need to learn to play with other children as well as alone or with you. Even babies and small children like other children's company, although at first they play alongside each other rather than together. Get together with other parents. It's worth doing because it helps your child get on with others.

You could start with something like a parent and toddler group or 'one o'clock club'. These can be great for energetic 18 month to three year olds, and give you a bit of relaxation and company. Ask other mothers or your health visitor about groups in your area. Or look on the clinic noticeboard, or in newsagents' or toy shop windows. Your local library may also have information, and may itself run story sessions for pre-school children.

Around the age of three, your child might go to a playgroup, nursery school or nursery class. All of these have a lot to offer; more organised play of different kinds, the chance to be with other children and make friends, probably space to run around in . . . Children also usually settle better at infant school if they've already had some experience of playing and learning with others.

Find out what is available in your area well in advance: there may be waiting lists.

Playgroups can be found in most areas. They vary in what they offer and how they are run. A small fee is usually charged. Sometimes you'll be able to leave your child, say for a couple of hours once or twice a week, so you can begin to get your child used to being away from you. Sometimes you'll be asked, or might want, to stay and help. Playgroups are often run by parents themselves.

To find out about local playgroups:

– ask your health visitor

— look on noticeboards at your clinic, health centre or library, or in newsagents' or toy shop windows

– ask your social services department (social work department in Scotland; health and social services board in Northern Ireland). They should have a list of local playgroups.

– contact the Pre-school Playgroups Association (address on page 94).

You might think about joining with other parents to start a playgroup yourselves. The Pre-school Playgroups Association can help (address on page 94).

A **nursery class** is part of an infant school. A **nursery school** is a separate school. Not every area has nursery schools or classes but it is worth finding out what is available. Ask your education department (see page

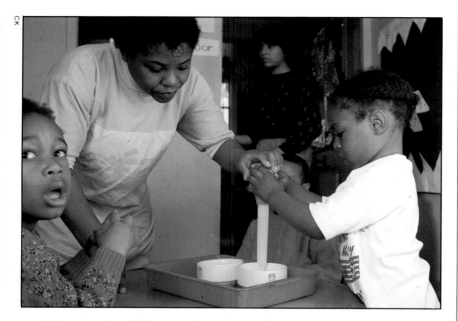

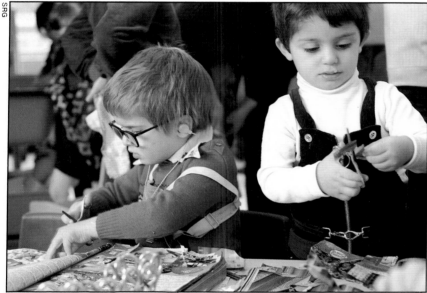

84), your health visitor, or other parents. Local authority nursery schools and classes are free.

Infant school starts sometime around the age of five. Legally, children must start infant school no later than the beginning of the school term following their 5th birthday. Some schools take children earlier, but it is important for your child to be ready. An early start isn't necessarily better.

Although parents are entitled to choose which school their child goes to, every school has a limit on the number of children it can take. So start looking at schools early, and check with the headteacher whether or not the school is likely to take your child. You can get a list of local schools from your education department (in your phone book under the name of your local authority).

FINDING A PLAYGROUP NURSERY OR INFANT SCHOOL

When considering a playgroup, nursery or infant school:

○ Go to see the group or school. See a few if you have a choice. Talk to the people in charge, look at what's going on, ask questions. You might, for example, want to ask:

– How many children there are in a group/school/class, and how many staff.
– How many of the staff are permanent and what their qualifications are.
– What your child's day would be like.
– What sort of discipline is used.
– What facilities there are, such as equipment, space to play outside, space to run around inside when the weather is bad, etc.
– Whether trips and visits are organised
– What effort is made to teach the children about different races, cultures and religions.

○ Trust your feelings. If you like the feel of a place, and the children seem happy and busy, that's a good sign. You know best the kind of place that will suit your child.

○ Talk to other parents whose children are at the group or school. Your health visitor may also be able to tell you about other parents' views and experiences.

○ Talk about ways of settling your child in happily. Staff may suggest ways of helping with this. At a playgroup or nursery school, you might, for example, stay with your child at first, then go away for longer and longer times. Some children are helped by this sort of gentle start; for others a clean break seems to work best. Some take to change and separation quite easily; others find it hard. Be prepared to give support and reassurance for quite some time if needed.

○ In some situations, *more* support and reassurance may be needed. For example, it may be that your child will be one of very few black children at a mainly white school – or one of very few white children. If you are facing this situation, talk to the school beforehand about the kind of difficulties that a different colour, culture or language might bring. Find out how the school will handle these, make suggestions yourself if you want to, and explain your child's needs. Talk with your child, too, in whatever way seems best.

Learning what has to be learnt

There always seem to be a lot of things you have to teach your child *not* to do. A day can be filled with 'don't do that' and 'stop doing that'. You'll find more about this sort of problem in Chapter 3. But from early on, there will also be things you want to teach your children to do for themselves, like using the potty, washing or dressing themselves, and so on. It's worth thinking about how you do it.

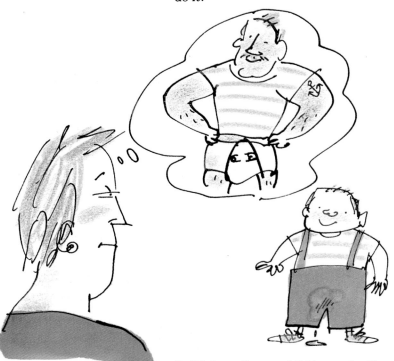

○ Wait until your child is ready. Forcing something too soon usually ends in failure. *You* get cross and upset, *your child* gets cross and upset, and the whole thing becomes impossible. On the other hand, some children never seem 'ready'. They seem content to go on wearing nappies, being dressed, being washed, for the rest of their lives. So:

○ Make it fun, make it interesting. This is the sort of advice that can make a tired, harassed parent despair. But if it's fun for your child, it's less likely to make you tired and harassed. And laughing about something can help your feelings as well as help your child.

○ Be encouraging. Showing you're pleased when something is achieved works better than telling your child off every time it's *not* achieved. So try to remember to say when you feel good about something your child has done or tried to do. Help him or her to feel good about it too.

○ Don't ask for perfection, or for instant success. It's safest to expect everything to take much longer than you'd hoped.

○ Set an example. Whatever it may look like, your child does want to be like you, do what you do. So seeing *you* wash in the bath, brush your teeth or use the toilet does help.

○ Avoid fuss and pressure. Be as low-key as you can. Once something gets blown up, it can take longer and be much more difficult for everybody.

○ Avoiding fuss and pressure doesn't mean you shouldn't be firm. Children need you to decide some things for them, and need you to stick to your decisions. They need some firm guidelines and limits. So try not to waver. You might start something like potty training, decide your child isn't ready, and give up for a while. That's fine. But a child who is in nappies one day, out the next, back in them the next, is bound to get confused.

○ For the same reason, it's important that everybody involved in looking after your child is teaching more or less the same things in more or less the same way. If you and your partner, or you and your childminder, do things very differently, your child won't learn so easily, and may well play you off against each other.

○ Do what's right for *your* child, for you and for the way you live. It doesn't matter what the child next door can or can't do. Don't compete; don't ask your child to compete.

All of this demands almost endless patience. And all parents have times when they run out of patience. See Chapter 3 for more about this.

"You think, if I handle this right, they'll learn, it'll get better. But you know sometimes it's just that you have to let time go by. Everything I wanted to happen happened in the end. Sometimes you can try too hard with them."

"It drives me mad. He's plenty old enough to use the toilet, but he won't have anything but the potty, and I'm running around all day emptying it. I had to leave him for a morning with my sister. So I took the potty and told her, you know, I'm sorry, but he won't use the toilet. And when I got back, it turned out he'd gone to the toilet every time, no fuss, nothing said or anything."

"Some things she wants to learn. Even if it's difficult, she wants to learn. With other things, she doesn't want to know. In fact, what she wants is to make a fuss. When it's like that, there's no way round it and I just have to put my foot down and get through it as quick as I can."

3. How do you cope?

"Why is it people seem to think it's an easy job looking after children? I did a lot of different jobs before I had children and I can tell you, none of them were as hard as this. None of them were as good. But none were so hard."

"The nicest thing anybody's ever said to me is, 'I think you're a good mother'. Often I think I'm a rotten mother. But just to be told you're doing a good job makes you better at it."

I don't have to be perfect!

Making life work

Being a parent is a very under-rated job, and very demanding. Unlike any other job, it goes on all the time. In fact, it's not just your job, it's your life. Even if you go out to work, you're still a full-time parent. So to feel all right in yourself, you really do need to feel you're doing it well.

But no parent 'does it well' all of the time. All parents have bad days, and most go through times when one bad day seems to follow another. Since you can't hand in your notice, or take a week off, you have to find some way of making life work.

"I've just stopped asking myself to be perfect. I've stopped trying so hard. You don't have to be perfect, and if you were, I don't think it would be that good for your child. People have to take me as they find me. That goes for the children, and it goes for people who drop in and find yesterday's washing up in the sink and a heap of dirty washing on the floor."

"My husband's mum is great in that, you know, she'll help me out with the kids. But she's got her own ideas about how they ought to be brought up and that, so we do have arguments. I think you've got to say, these are the things I'm going to stick out for, and these are the things I'm not going to bother about. But there've got to be some things where what *you* say and what *you* feel goes. And then you can stop caring – or arguing – about the rest."

"I get guilty if I take time for myself, and I get angry if I *don't* have time for myself. So I say, 'Right. You let me do this, and then I'll do that with you.' I did it when he was a baby and didn't have any choice. And I do it now when he's old enough to understand."

"At the beginning, I think I thought nobody could do it but me. It had to be me, all the time. But you'd have to be superhuman to live like that with small children. You've got to share the work, and you've got to ask other people to help you out."

Getting on with each other

Making life work isn't just a matter of getting the jobs done. It's not just a matter of surviving. You also want your child to be happy and contented, not least because that helps *you* feel happy and contented.

Often this is the hardest part – to cope when your child is awkward or moody or difficult and still to stay friends and enjoy the good bits that come in between.

"The smallest thing can turn into an argument. A whole morning can be spoilt, just because of some stupid thing like brushing hair, or insisting she says 'please', or saying we can't go to the playground because it's raining, or, you know, things that come out of nowhere."

"I think what's so wearing is that it all depends on mood. Not just their mood, but mine too. And you have to hide your feelings away so much, and they just let theirs out. If they want to lie down and cry because their favourite T-shirt's in the wash or you won't buy them something at the shops, they just do it. And when they do it in front of other people, that's awful."

When you're tired or in a bad mood, or when your child is tired or in a bad mood, it can be hard to get on together and get through the day. You can end up arguing non-stop. Even the smallest thing can make you angry. If you go out to work, it's especially disappointing if the short time you've got to spend with your child is spoilt by arguments.

Moods apart, most children also go through patches of being difficult or awkward over certain things – dressing, or eating, or going to bed at night. Knowing that it makes you cross or upset probably makes them still more difficult. And you become more and more tense, and less and less able to cope.

At the end of a bad day or a tough week, it's worth thinking about what you can do, for your sake as well as your child's.

○ Change your routine. Do things at different times. An argument that always happens at one time of day may not happen at another. And do the difficult things when your child is least tired or most co-operative. For example, try dressing your child after breakfast rather than before; have lunch earlier – or later. And so on.

○ Give your child either/or choices. Not 'What would you like to wear today?' but 'Do you want this pullover or that one?' or 'Shall we do this now, or that?'

○ Distract your child from whatever you know is going to cause a problem. The *second* your child starts being difficult, or even before, find something interesting to look at or talk about or do. Put on an act. Create a diversion. Best of all, find something to laugh about.

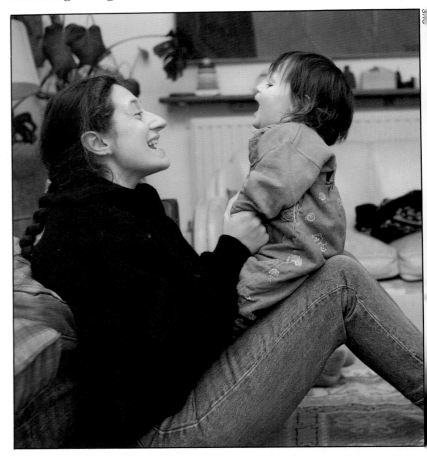

○ Ask yourself whether whatever you're about to tell your child off about really matters. Sometimes it does, sometimes it doesn't. Having arguments about certain things can get to be a habit.

○ Don't expect too much. Of course you want your child to try, and to achieve new things, be well-behaved, and do as he or she is told. But it's very easy to demand more than your child can give and then find yourself being cross because your demands aren't met. It's asking a lot of you, but in the end it's probably best *not* to expect good behaviour for long periods of time or when your child is tired; *not* to expect your child to listen to, let alone do, what you say the first or even the second time you say it; *not* to expect your child to be tidy; and so on and so on. If it's all right for you to be a less than perfect parent, then it's all right for your child to be less than perfect too. It's just hard to live with sometimes.

○ Try to notice the good things. If you feel good about something your child does, say so. It's good for him or her, and it makes you feel more positive too.

○ When you *do* have arguments, enjoy making up afterwards. And if you've lost your temper because you're tired or upset, say you're sorry. It will help you both feel better.

The way you feel

Parents spend a lot of time coping with their children's feelings. But you have to cope with the way *you* feel too. This is at least half the battle.

"I know often they wind me up so much I'll tell them off for nothing. It doesn't do me any good, and it doesn't do them any good either. I try to *make* myself ignore things, and that works quite well. None of it matters nearly as much as I think it does when I'm wound up and tense. And if I can say to myself, 'It doesn't matter', then I don't get wound up so much in the first place."

(A father) "When I was working, I used to think it must be easy being at home all day. You know, just the kids and you, and you can suit yourself really. I'm at home all day now, being out of a job, and that's when you begin to see what it's all about. But the thing is, when one of you has had enough, then the other can take over, and you get a breathing space."

"Sometimes I will smack her because she's done something really bad or really dangerous. But other times I know I want to smack her just because of the way I'm feeling, and after, I'll feel bad about it. When it's like that, I just walk away. If John's at home, I'll ask him to take over. And if I'm on my own, I just go into another room and count to ten."

"I'll do anything rather than hit him. I'll hit cushions, the wall, I'll shout at the top of my voice. Sometimes you've got to get rid of it all somehow, but I don't want him to even see that, let alone get the brunt of it."

"I feel like I'm trapped. Inside my own four walls, that's when it can get bad. So I put her in the buggy and walk. It doesn't matter what the weather's like, or where I go, so long as I get outside. I used to feel, you know, it's too much effort to get out, with all the dressing up and the rest. But if you think like that, you never go out and it all gets on top of you without you ever realising it."

"My mum's my best friend really. It sounds old-fashioned, but she is. You can say anything to your mum. I can have a good moan to her and she doesn't think anything the worse of me. I can let off steam."

"When it gets too much, I drop everything and get out. I go and see people, find somebody to talk to. I'm a different person when I'm with other people."

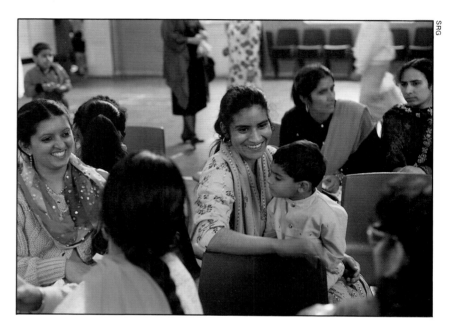

SRG

It does help to talk and be with other people, especially other parents. It's often true that 'only parents understand'. A lot look very calm and capable from the outside (and you may do too), but alone at home most get frustrated and angry at times.

If you don't already know other parents living nearby, look at page 87 for how to find out about local groups. Groups don't suit everybody, but at the very least they are a way of making friends. And a group which is run by parents specially for parents can often give you more than friends who haven't got children the same age.

Sometimes, whatever you do, feelings of anger and frustration get out of control. Then it's vital to get support. Talk to your health visitor, and/or contact one of the parent support organisations listed on page 94. Some of these organisations, like the National Society for the Prevention of Cruelty to Children (NSPCC), and Parentline and Parents Anonymous (which run telephone helplines), have been set up especially to help parents under stress by people who understand what the effects can be.

When you're on your own

"The thing is, everything's on your shoulders. When you have to decide something, you know, like whether or not to take him to the doctor, or even everyday small things, there's nobody to share that with. There are so many things it's useful to talk about, and if you're on your own, you can't. If there's a crisis, you're on you own."

"It's less stressful being your own boss. There's more satisfaction somehow, more achievement. There's no-one to disagree with, no conflict over discipline, no competition with other adults. And it means you've got a stronger bond, you're better friends."

"There's no company in the evenings. That's almost the hardest part. You put the kids to bed at night and that's it."

Bringing up children alone can bring huge pleasures, huge rewards. The problems it can also bring may not be so very different from problems faced by two-parent families. But problems can look and feel different when you're alone, and are often harder to solve.

Getting support, finding friends, making time for yourself, are often more important but much more difficult when you're on your own. Possibilities may be:

○ Local groups. (Mother and baby, parent and toddler groups, and so on.) Ask your health visitor what's going on locally, and look through the list of parent support organisations on page 94 – many run local groups.

○ Gingerbread – a self-help organisation run by and for one-parent families (address on page 94). It has local groups around the country. Through these groups you can meet parents in similar situations to your own. And you can often help each other out as well as supporting each other generally.

○ A 'swap' arrangement with another parent so you get, say, a morning off one week, look after the children the next.

○ A playgroup or nursery school/class for your child when he or she is old enough. See page 32.

○ Asking someone to babysit for the odd evening. When you can't return evening babysitting, it can be difficult to get an evening out. But if you can think of anybody at all whom you'd trust and who might help out, there's nothing lost by *asking*. You may be able to repay with daytime babysitting. Or you could take your child to someone else's house for an evening and have their child back in return. Older children could perhaps stay the night with a friend or relative. The important thing is to look at possibilities and have the courage to ask for help. It won't do you or your child any good if you never get out alone.

Money and housing are often problems for lone parents. Look at 'Rights and benefits' (pages 89-93) to check you are claiming all you are entitled to. See pages 84-5 for information about help with housing problems. If you are working, or thinking of it, see pages 81-92 for information about child care.

The National Council for One Parent Families (address on page 94) offers free advice to lone parents – for example, on rights and benefits.

Coping with a second baby

"When you've got the one, you don't know how easy it is. Once you've got the two of them, it's much more than twice the work. At the beginning, when the second's only a baby still, that's the most difficult time of all."

"When I only had one, if he had a tantrum, I found I could ignore it and stay fairly calm. Now, with the two of them, if I try to ignore anything, it turns into a full-scale war."

"I feel split in two. They pull me in different directions the whole time and it's almost impossible to do right by both of them. What's right for the baby is wrong for my older one, and the same the other way round. I love them both, but there doesn't seem any way of showing them that, or of being fair."

Coping with two children is very different from coping with one and it can be tough at first, especially if your first child isn't very old. So far as the baby goes, you've got more experience and probably more confidence, which helps. But the work more than doubles, and dividing your time and attention can be a strain.

It's not unusual for the birth of a second baby to alter your feelings towards your first child. It would be strange if it didn't. At first, you may feel that you are somehow not

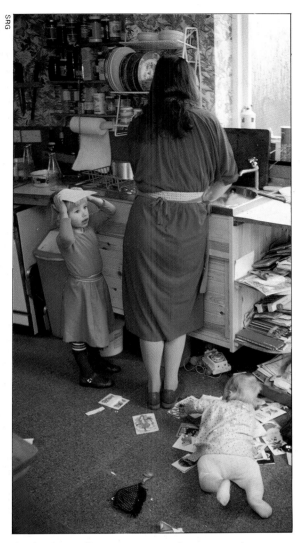

SRG

some time alone together, so your older one doesn't feel pushed out.

○ Older children don't always find babies very lovable, but they do often find them interesting. You may be able to encourage this. There's a lot you can say and explain about babies, and children like to be given facts. Talk about what your older one was like and did as a baby. Get out the old toys and photos. And try to make looking after and playing with the baby a good game – without expecting too much.

○ Feeds are often difficult. An older child may well feel left out and jealous. Find something for him or her to do, or make feeds a time for a story or a chat. With help, some older children can bottle feed a baby themselves.

○ Be prepared for your older child to go back to baby behaviour for a time – wanting a bottle, wetting pants, wanting to be carried. It's hard, but don't always refuse requests, and try not to get angry.

There *will* be jealousy and resentment, shown one way or another, sooner or later. You can only do so much. If you and your partner, or you and a grandparent or friend, can sometimes give each other time alone with each child, you won't feel so constantly pulled in different directions.

loving your first one as much or enough. Some parents say they feel very protective towards the baby and 'go off' the older one for a while. It simply takes time to adjust to being a bigger family and loving more than one child.

Your older child, no matter what his or her age, has to adjust too. You can probably help with this, and that will help you.

○ Try to keep on as many of the old routines and activities as you can – like going to playgroup, going to visit friends, telling a bedtime story. This may not be easy in the early weeks, but it gives reassurance.

○ Don't expect your older child to be pleased with the baby or feel the way you do. It's lovely if the pleasure *is* shared, but best not to expect it.

○ Do expect an older child to be more demanding and to want more and need more of you. Someone like a granny can often help by giving the older one time. But try to give some special attention yourself, and have

Twins

Parents who only have one child often think that having two together is much the same sort of experience, but doubled. If you have twins, you'll know different. Caring for twins, or more, is very different to caring for one child, or even caring for two of different ages. There's certainly a lot more work, and often you have to find different ways of doing things.

You need as much support as you can get. If you haven't already got that support from family and friends, or even if you have, you need to go out and look for it. The Twins and Multiple Births Association (address on page 94) offers a lot of helpful information, including information about local Twins Clubs. Through these clubs you can meet other parents whose experiences are like yours, and get support and practical advice. Often you can get secondhand equipment too, such as twin prams and buggies.

Dealing with difficult behaviour

People have very different ideas about good and bad behaviour. What is bad behaviour to you may be accepted as normal by other parents, and vice versa. Sometimes it's a matter of a particular family's rules. Sometimes it's more to do with circumstances. It's much harder to put up with mess if you haven't got much space, or with noise if the walls are thin.

"The thing is that what you have to ask of them isn't always what you'd want to ask. It's how things are. My husband works nights and he has to sleep mornings. There's no way round that. If the children are noisy, he can't sleep."

People also react to their children's behaviour very differently. Some are tougher than others; some are more patient than others; and so on. It's not just a matter of how you decide to be. It's also how you are as a person.

"You get a lot of advice about how to handle your children and I think, because a lot of the time you feel very unsure of yourself, you get to think that there's a 'right' way. When you read something, or get a bit of advice, or see somebody handling their child a certain way, you forget to stop and think, you know, 'Is that me?'"

It's best to set your own rules to fit the way you live and the way you are. And it's best to deal with your child's behaviour *your* way.

But for all parents there are times when their children's behaviour gets them down or really worries them. There are times when nothing you do seems to work. What do you do then?

Understanding difficult behaviour

Try to step back and do some thinking.

○ **Is it really a problem?**   In other words, is it a problem that you feel you *must* do something about; or might it be better to just live with it for a while? Sometimes it is trying to *do* something about a certain sort of behaviour that changes it from something that's irritating for you into a real problem for your child. But if a problem is causing you and your child distress, or upsetting family life, then you do need to do something about it.

It's also worth asking yourself whether your child's behaviour is a problem in your eyes, or only in other people's. Sometimes some kind of behaviour that you can happily ignore, or at any rate aren't worried about, is turned into a problem by other people's comments.

○ **Is there a reason?**   There usually is, and it's worth trying to work it out before you do anything. Think about:

– the sort of person your child is. You'll know your child's character and may be able to see that a certain sort of behaviour fits that character. For example, if your child is quite emotional, something like night-time waking and bad dreams are not so hard to understand. And being tough may not be the right answer.

– what your child has to cope with. At certain times especially, small children have a lot to cope with. A lot is asked of them, there's a lot they can't or aren't allowed to do. And any change in their lives, like the birth of a new baby, moving house, a change of childminder, starting playgroup, or even a much smaller change, can be a big event. Sometimes they show the stress they are feeling by being difficult.

– the way you are, or the family is, at present. Children react to family upset, and to the moods of people close to them. If you yourself are worried about something, if you're under stress, if there's some sort of family tension, your child is more than likely to pick that up. He or she may then become difficult at just the time when you feel least able to cope.

If a problem is more yours than your child's, don't blame yourself for that. But try not to blame your child either.

– the way you've handled a problem. Sometimes the way you've dealt with a problem in the past can catch you out. For example, you may have taken your child into bed with you when he or she was small because that was the only way of getting a night's sleep. For you, that was the right answer *then*. But now your child won't sleep alone.

○ Think too about **how you react** when your child is difficult. If a tantrum brings attention (even angry attention), or night-time waking means company and a cuddle, then maybe your child has a good reason for behaving that way. You may need to try to give more attention at other times, and less attention to the problem.

○ Think about **the times when the bad behaviour happens**. Is it, for example, when your child is tired, hungry, over-excited, frustrated, bored?

If you can think around your child's behaviour a bit and begin to understand it, you're more likely to find a right answer. And even if you can't find an answer, you'll probably cope better.

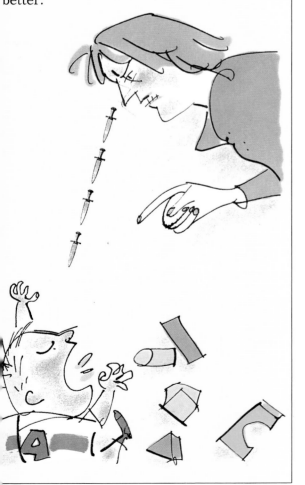

How you deal with it

Do what feels right – for your child, for you and for the family. If you do anything you don't believe in, or anything you feel isn't right, it's far less likely to work. Children usually know when you don't really mean something.

Don't give up too quickly   Once you've decided to do something, give it a fair trial. You may want to set a time limit: a week, or a month, or whatever seems right. But stick to your limit. Very few solutions work overnight.

It's easier to stick at something if you have someone to support you. Get help from your partner, a friend, another parent, your health visitor or doctor. At the very least, it is good to have someone to talk to about progress – or lack of it.

Try to be consistent
Children need to know where they stand. If you react to their behaviour one way one day, a different way the next, it's confusing. It is also important that everyone close to your child deals with the problem in the same way.

Try not to overreact   This is very hard. When your child does something annoying not just once but time after time, your own feelings of anger or frustration are bound to build up. But if you become very tense and wound up over a problem, you can end up taking your feelings out on your child. The whole situation can get out of control. You don't have to hide the way you feel. It would be inhuman not to show irritation and anger sometimes. But hard as it is, try to keep a sense of proportion. Once you've said what needs to be said and let your feelings out, try to leave it at that. Move on to other things – that you can both enjoy or feel good about. And look for other ways of coping with your feelings (see page 37).

Talk   Children don't have to be able to talk back to understand. And understanding might help. So it could be worth explaining why, for example, you don't want them in your bed, or why you get cross about something.

Hold on to what's good about your child, about your relationship, about you as a parent. When a child is being really difficult, it can come to dominate everything. That doesn't help anybody. What *can* help is to say (or show) when you feel good about something.

Rewards sometimes work. You might want to promise something like a special outing, for example, if your child manages to do something. But rewards like this are best used as a last resort, and only every now and then. If they're used too often, they lose their value, and they can become a kind of trap. You can end up bargaining over everything.

Rewards can also put pressure on a child, when maybe what's needed is to take the pressure off. If you promise a treat in advance and your child doesn't manage to 'earn' it, it can cause a lot of disappointment and difficulty. Giving a reward *after* something has been achieved, rather than promising it beforehand, is less risky. And after all, a hug is a reward.

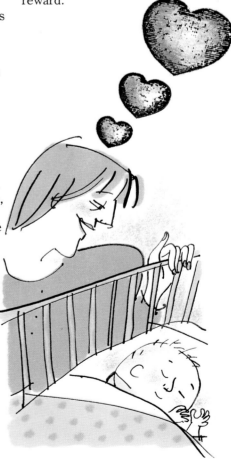

Particular problems

Not all these ideas for coping with particular problems will suit you. Look for what you think is right for you and your child and for what's possible in your situation. All the ideas have worked for some families. Remember that most take time to work.

Problems with food

Refusing to eat, or eating very little

○ Don't force your child to eat. There's usually no need to worry about whether your child is getting enough to eat. Most eat when they're hungry, though maybe not what you want them to eat – see 'Being choosy', next column. And a child can be perfectly fit and healthy on remarkably little. So long as your child *is* fit and healthy, and growing and gaining weight, don't fuss. If you are worried, talk to your health visitor or doctor.

○ If food is refused, or just picked at for a long time, call an end to the meal. Do it calmly and not in anger, no matter what time and effort you've put into the cooking.

○ Put less on your child's plate.

○ Try to make meals enjoyable and not just about eating. Chat about things other than food.

○ Games can help but are also a bit dangerous. Sometimes a game to do with eating, like lorries taking food to the depot, can help a child concentrate on eating. Sometimes games like this become the same as force feeding.

○ If you know other children of the same age who are good eaters, have them to lunch or tea. A good example sometimes works – so long as you don't go on about how good the other children are.

○ Ask another adult whom your child likes to eat with you. Sometimes a child will eat for, say, a grandparent, without any fuss at all. It may be only one meal out of many, but it could break a habit.

○ Try limiting snacks and drinks between meals. You may be able to cut down by promising snacks at certain times and finding other distractions. But also ask yourself whether meals matter all that much. They do in some families, but not in all. If you don't mind your child not eating 'proper meals', a different solution may be to make between-meal snacks more nutritious.

Being choosy

○ Give the foods your child *will* eat and forget about the others for a while. Usually you can manage a bit of variety, even if it's the same variety every day. If your child eats say beans and fish fingers, bread and, hopefully, a bit of fruit, every day for a month, it will seem odd to you but isn't in fact such a bad diet. A drink of milk, if your child will have it, will make the menu a bit healthier.

○ Let your child eat with other children, especially those who eat anything and everything. Children who aren't very good about new foods will sometimes try them if they see other children eating them. Don't press – just let your child watch.

○ Carry on eating the variety of foods *you* like to eat. It may seem easiest to cook only what your child will eat, but that's not going to be much of a diet for you, and your child will never get a chance to have a change of mind and try something out. Try to find meals where you can pick out one or two things your child will eat, and where you can eat the lot.

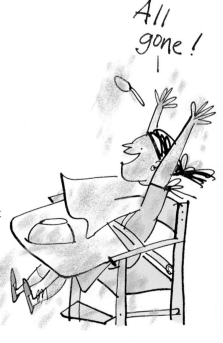

All gone!

Sleep problems

Trouble at bedtime

Not all parents feel it's important to get their children off to bed at a certain time or in a certain way. In some families, children simply go to bed when they're ready – or at the same time as their parents. Some parents are happy to cuddle their children off to sleep every night. But others want bedtime to be more organised and early enough to give their children a long sleep and give them some child-free time.

○ Of course, you stand a better chance of success at bedtime if your child is really tired, both mentally and physically. Try to get outside at least once in the day – and not just to give *you* exercise pushing the buggy. Get your child together with other children; they are good at tiring each other out. Find *new* activities; a change is often tiring, and something like going swimming can work the odd miracle. Sometimes it works to cut out an afternoon sleep, once you feel your child is old enough.

Some children never seem to get tired and can keep going longer than you. Just do the best you can.

○ Go through the same routine every night – something like: bath, games in the bath, story, quiet time to talk, sleep. Invent as much as you can to make it fun, and try to make it a time when you give time and attention. But wind down, and don't let the ending go on and on. Be firm and make it clear that at a certain point the day must and does come to an end.

○ Children who won't be left, or have to be cuddled to sleep, can sometimes be weaned off it in stages. One week you sit by the bed holding hands. The next week you sit close by but don't hold hands. The next you sit further away. And so on. Don't talk if you can avoid it.

○ Leave a light on. Perhaps a ceiling or bedside light with a low bulb. Or try a dimmer switch. You can also buy glow plugs. They fit into an ordinary socket and give a very low light.

○ Try to get your child to go to sleep with a toy or some kind of comforter instead of with you.

○ Leave the radio or a tape on – quietly.

○ Make your child's cot or bed into a special place with pictures, mobiles etc.

○ Leave books and toys around. Some children settle better if left to play for a while, perhaps in a slightly dimmed light. Others wind themselves up again this way, and then it is better to take toys *out* of the room, perhaps leaving one favourite, quiet toy and a book.

○ If your child cries or makes a fuss when you leave the room, wait ten minutes, go back, re-settle your child the same way as usual, go away again. Repeat this as often as you need or can bear, but be firm. You are saying, 'I'm here, I haven't gone away, I love you, but it's time for sleep.'

○ If you become desperate and your feelings are getting out of control, you could try leaving your child to cry or shout. Don't go back – sit it out. This is no good for older children. They will simply walk out of the room and come to find you. You can't shut them in. And for younger children, you do have to be desperate to try it as some will cry for hours. For some families it has worked. But if you find (say, after a few days of agony) that it isn't working for you, give up.

In the past, drugs were often prescribed for children with sleep problems. They are now rarely used. This is partly because their effects are a bit uncertain, and partly because they are not a long-term answer. If you have grown desperate and your child's problem is very bad, it's important to get help. Your doctor may prescribe a drug which will at least give you a break for a few nights, but you will need to talk about other solutions too. Another possibility is to find someone else to take over for the odd night, or even to have your child to stay. You will cope better if you can catch up on some sleep yourself.

Waking in the night

It's normal for babies and toddlers to wake in the night. Up to a half of all children under five go through periods of night-waking. The problem is really your own lack of sleep. For a time, the best way to cope may be to accept disturbed nights as best you can, getting as much sleep and as much support as you possibly can during the day.

○ If your child is waking from fear or bad dreams, try talking about it. Try and find the reasons (shadows? something seen on television? some family upset?) and sort them out if you can. (Children don't normally wake from bad dreams much before two and a half to three years old.)

○ For children who have their own bedrooms, leave a light on, leave books and toys about. Some children will wake, play for a while, and get themselves off to sleep again. You could leave a drink of water by the bed.

○ If the reason isn't fear, then try to be firm and fairly brief. Don't take your child out of the room. Don't start long conversations, stories or games. Try to show that night-time is for sleeping, not company.

○ Take your child into your bed. Some parents like doing this anyway. If you have two children sharing one bedroom, and one is likely to wake the other, it can be the only answer. You may worry that it will become a habit, and it's true that it may. But if it's a way of getting some sleep, that may be all that matters. It's possible to move some children back to their own beds once they've fallen asleep again.

○ If your child sleeps in a bed, you could get in for a while, until your child is asleep again.

○ Some of the suggestions under 'Trouble at bedtime' may help.

Wet children

Most children are more or less dry by day by the age of three, whether you've trained them or not. But lots go on wetting at night for some time after this. Lots of parents search for some way of training their children to be dry as early as possible, really because it means less work. Most parents with older children would say that the only thing you can do about wetting, either by day or by night, is put up with it until it stops.

(For information about potty training, and the development of bladder control, see page 28.)

○ Take the pressure off. This might mean giving up the potty and going back to nappies for a while, or just living a wet life and not letting it get you or your child down.

○ Show you're pleased and help your child to be pleased when he or she uses the potty or toilet or manages to stay dry, even for a short time. Be gentle about accidents. You need to explain that it is not what's wanted. But do your best not to show irritation or to nag. Once a child becomes worried, the problem often gets worse.

○ Limit drinks a bit. Many children go through a stage of demanding a lot to drink. Try to limit drinks to certain times and make them 'special' rather than routine. Or give just a few drinks of juice (if that is what is demanded), and water in between. Most children drink less if it is only water that is offered. Some children drink for comfort or just for something to do. Other distractions, or using another sort of 'comforter', might help.

○ For **bed-wetting**, make sure you don't give too much to drink before bed. Show how pleased you are when your child manages a dry night. You might want to give a reward (see page 41). If the problem goes on, try getting your child up and putting him or her on the potty or toilet – say, at the time you go to bed. Most aren't disturbed by this and settle again very quickly. Do all you can not to be angry. Many four to five year olds do wet the bed. It's often easiest to leave them in nappies at night. It saves washing sheets.

Constipation, and 'soiling'

○ Make sure your child isn't frightened. Reassure. Let your child be with you when you go to the toilet. And try to be as relaxed as you can be about the problem.

○ Make sure your child eats plenty of fibre – from wholemeal bread, chappattis, wholegrain breakfast cereals, fruit and vegetables. Baked beans, frozen peas and sweetcorn are good sources of fibre often liked by children. Also give lots to drink – clear drinks rather than milk. All this will help to prevent constipation.

Once a child becomes constipated, stools can become hard and painful to pass out. The pain means the child holds back even more, becomes more constipated, has more pain, and so on. It's important to stop this spiral. Giving a mild laxative may help. Ask your health visitor or doctor to recommend a suitable one. If it doesn't solve the problem quickly, talk to your doctor.

○ Constipation and/or soiling pants sometimes happen when a child is upset about something. All you may be able to do is help your child feel as happy and secure as possible day to day, and wait for the problem to pass. But if it continues and you're worried, talk to your health visitor or doctor.

Tempers, tantrums

Tantrums may start around 18 months, are common around two, much less common at four. Twenty per cent of two year olds have temper tantrums at least twice a day. One reason is that around this age children often want to express themselves more than they are able. They feel frustrated, and the frustration comes out as a tantrum. Once a child can talk more, tantrums often lessen.

○ Tantrums tend to happen when children are tired or hungry. Sleep or food might be the answer.

○ Otherwise, try to work out the reason and tackle that. It may be frustration. It may be something like jealousy. More time and attention, and being extra loving (even when your child is not so lovable), can help.

○ Even if you can't be sure of the reason, try to understand and accept the anger your child is feeling. You probably feel the same way yourself very often. If you think about that, you may be better able to accept your child's feelings.

○ When a tantrum is starting, try to find instant distraction. Work at this for all you're worth. Find something to look at – out of the window, for example. Make yourself sound really surprised and interested in it.

○ Try sitting the tantrum out. Don't lose your temper or shout back. Ignore the looks you get from people around you. Stay as calm as you can, try not to get involved, but don't give in. If you've said 'no', don't change your mind and say 'yes' just to end the tantrum. If you do change your mind, your child will think that tantrums pay. For the same reason, don't buy your way out with sweets or treats. If you're at home, you could try walking away into another room.

○ Tantrums often seem to happen in shops. This can be really embarrassing, and embarrassment makes it extra hard to cope and stay calm. Keep shopping trips short. You could start by going out to buy one or two things only, and then build up from there. Once you've managed one quick trip without trouble, you're beginnning to make progress.

○ Some parents find it helps to hold their child, quite firmly, until the tantrum passes. This usually only works when your child is more upset than angry, and when you yourself are feeling calm and able to talk gently and reassuringly.

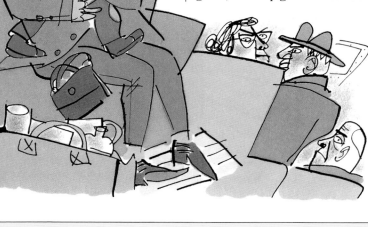

There's always a limit to what you can do when your child is being especially difficult in some way. Very often, the problem just disappears with time and you have to hold on until it does. Other parents can help you do that. It's by meeting and talking with other parents that you find out that you are not the only one whose child is difficult in some way, and not the only one who finds it hard to cope. Many of the organisations listed on page 94 (such as the National Childbirth Trust, Home-Start, Parent Network and others) run local groups or schemes.
  If you become very worried about your child's behaviour, if you can't cope or live with it, or feel it's gone on for too long, get help. Contact one of the organisations listed on page 94 and/or talk to your health visitor, clinic doctor or family doctor. They can often suggest something helpful, and support *you*. You can, if you wish, be referred to a specialist for help. If you've got a special problem, it's right to get special help.

Hitting, biting, kicking, fighting . . .

○ Don't hit, bite or kick back. It makes behaving like that seem all right. You can still make it clear that it hurts.

○ Talk. Children often go through patches of insecurity or upset and let their feelings out by being aggressive – at playgroup, for example. If by talking you can find out what is worrying your child, you may be able to help.

○ Children who are being aggressive aren't so easy to love. But extra love may be what is needed. Try to show how much you love your child, even though you don't love the way he or she is behaving.

○ Help your child let his or her feelings out. Running around, throwing themselves about, screaming and screeching, hitting cushions and so on, all as part of a game, can help get rid of tension.

Overactive children

Many parents say their children are 'hyperactive'. In fact real hyperactivity is rare. But quite a lot of children are extremely active, restless and difficult to manage. And an overactive child, or even a 'normally' active child, will be much harder to handle if, for example, you live in a small flat.

○ Keep to a daily routine as much as you can. Routine can be important for restless, difficult children. Routine may also help *you* stay calmer and stand up better to the strain.

○ Make giving your child time and attention a part of the routine. In different ways, your child may be demanding your attention most of the day, if not most of the night as well. A lot of the time you will have to say 'no'. This is easier to say, and may be easier for your child to accept, if there are certain times each day when you do give all your attention to your child.

○ It's often no good even expecting an overactive, difficult child to sit still at meals or behave well in a supermarket. Avoid difficult situations as much as you can – by keeping shopping trips short, for example. And try lowering your expectations. Start by asking your child to be still, or controlled, or to concentrate, for very short times. Then gradually build up.

○ Try to get out every day you can to a place where your child can run around and really let go. Go to a park, or a playground, or whatever safe, open space there is. Find ways of helping your child burn off energy.

(For information about the possible link between overactivity and food additives, see page 50)

4. Children's health

Feeding the family

"Yes, I want my kids to eat the right sort of things. But wanting it is one thing and doing it, or getting them to do it, is something else altogether. Mostly what one will eat the other won't. The only things I know they'll both eat are things like chips and sausages. Family meals almost always mean one of them making a fuss. You can make something for them that takes twice as long as sausages or whatever, and you end up putting it all in the bin."

"I've got 15 quid a week for the food and that's it. You don't get much choice for 15 quid. I know what I'd *like* to give the family to eat, and I know what I can afford to give them, and they're nothing like the same."

"When you go shopping, your mind's on anything but the shopping. You can't stop and think. You grab what you can and get out quick."

"Everybody knows that sweets aren't good. But they love them. And the fact is, it's a pleasure to me to treat them. All the same, I'd rather not be forced into giving treats when I don't want to, like at the supermarket check-out."

"There was a time when I could have listed the number of things she'd eat on the fingers of one hand. And she made so much fuss if I tried to get her to eat anything else, I just gave it up. Food isn't worth that much unhappiness. Anyway, somehow or other she did start to eat other things. You know, she'd be given something by her gran, and just because it was her gran, she'd eat it, and come home demanding the very thing she'd refused for months."

"It's difficult to give them healthy food because of the money. But some of the stuff that's not healthy costs most of all. Like sweets. And there are things you can do. Like beans and lentils and things are cheap and you can store them. And I slice up fruit and share it between the kids so it goes further."

Most children make a fuss about, or just refuse to eat, some foods. And it's a fact that very often the foods that are refused are the ones that are 'healthy'. If it was 'healthy' to eat a lot of biscuits, healthy eating wouldn't be a problem in families with small children.

Fussiness isn't the only problem. Shopping and cooking are hard work when you have small children. Food isn't cheap, and often the money won't stretch. And a lot of children seem to store up their worst behaviour especially for mealtimes.

Still, you don't have to aim at perfection. You're only aiming at feeding the family in a reasonably healthy way. Whatever the problems, you can probably do enough to make sure you all get more or less what you need.

Check the way your family eats against the information here. There may be changes you can make that won't put up your weekly food bill but will make you all a bit healthier.

Until they are five, children need a relatively high amount of calories and nutrients to ensure good growth. If they are eating a varied diet, some of the changes suggested for reducing fat and increasing fibre can be introduced slowly between two and five.

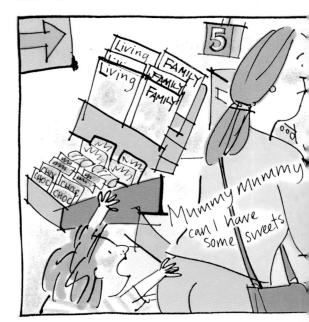

What's needed?

Variety

What's needed most of all is variety in what you eat.

'Variety' means, in the space of a day or even a week, eating different types of food: fruit and vegetables as well as meat, fish or pulses (peas, beans, lentils); dairy foods as well as bread, chappattis, rice or pasta; and so on. If you can eat a variety of foods, you'll almost certainly get all the nutrients you need.

If your child is choosy, try to make as varied a menu as you can from the foods he or she will eat. It's usually possible to give even very choosy children some variety. You may find you go through stages of giving the *same* variety day after day, but this need not matter. Gradually, over time, you'll be able to add new foods.

"I do feel, you know, I wish she'd eat that. But I'm resigned to it, really. Because even getting her to *try* things is hard. So I just serve up the same old things, and it's a fairly good mix, so why worry? I mean, she does eat different sorts of food. She eats baked beans, she loves bread, she'll drink milk. Potatoes and cheese always go down okay. She has orange juice and apples, bananas sometimes. There's nothing wrong with that."

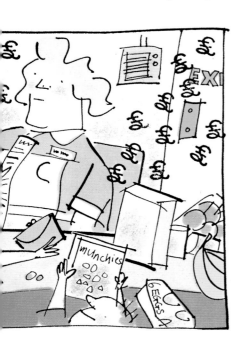

Not too much fat

Fat contains a lot of calories. Calories are a measurement of the amount of energy given by foods – and children need energy to grow. But if they eat more than their body needs, they may become overweight.

Too much fat, especially **saturated fat** is also linked with a higher risk of coronary heart disease because it builds up the level of cholesterol in the arteries. The arteries can become blocked, causing a heart attack. This process can begin in childhood. So, for children as well as adults, it's best not to eat too much fat, and especially saturated fat. Saturated fats are found in animal fats; in meat products; in hard margarine and some vegetable oils (such as coconut and palm oil); and in many bought foods like cakes, biscuits and chocolate. Dairy foods like milk and cheese also contain saturated fats but they are good sources of calcium, protein and vitamins. Lower fat versions are also rich in most of these nutrients – so why not try them?

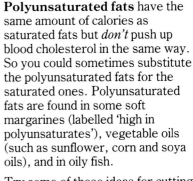

Polyunsaturated fats have the same amount of calories as saturated fats but *don't* push up blood cholesterol in the same way. So you could sometimes substitute the polyunsaturated fats for the saturated ones. Polyunsaturated fats are found in some soft margarines (labelled 'high in polyunsaturates'), vegetable oils (such as sunflower, corn and soya oils), and in oily fish.

Try some of these ideas for cutting down on fat:

○ Grill or bake instead of frying food. If you do fry, use a polyunsaturated oil like soya, sunflower or corn oil.

○ Skim fat off fatty meat dishes, like mince or curry, during cooking.

○ Choose fish or poultry without the skin. The skin is the fattiest part.

○ Trim the visible fat off red meat.

○ Use pulses and other vegetables instead of, or to boost small amounts of meat in stews, casseroles etc.

○ Use low-fat spread or a margarine high in polyunsaturates rather than butter, hard margarine or ordinary soft margarine.

○ Use a lower-fat cheese like one of the low-fat Cheddars, Edam or cottage cheese.

Milk. It's a good idea to carry on with breast or infant formula in the first year. You can begin to use cow's milk for mixing foods after six months as long as there is no family history of allergy. When you decide to introduce it, use whole pasteurised milk because this contains the calories and vitamins that a very young child needs. Semi-skimmed milk can be introduced into the diet after two years if you're sure your child is a good eater. Skimmed milk is not recommended for children under the age of five years.

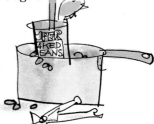

Not much sugar

You don't *need* sugar at all. It contains no nutrients, only calories. Since you get calories from everything you eat, you don't need any extra. Sugar also leads to tooth decay (see page 50).

Besides the sugar you use in cooking or add to food or drink, there's a lot of sugar in foods you buy; biscuits, cake, jam, honey, fruit tinned in syrup, sweetened fruit yogurts, sweets, chocolate, squash and fizzy drinks, and a lot of processed food. It can turn up in unexpected places – tomato ketchup, for example.

Brown sugar and honey are no better for you than white sugar.

"A lot of it is habit. I mean, if your children have never had sugar on their cereal in the morning, then they don't expect it. But then you mustn't have it either. The thing is that I like sweet things myself. In fact, at the moment, the more I get, the more I want to eat biscuits and that sort of thing. But if I eat them, the children eat them. The only answer is not to buy them in the first place."

Very few families either can or want to cut out sugar altogether. A lot *do* manage to cut down – and save money in the process.

○ Give children unsweetened fruit juice (diluted is cheaper and better for teeth), milk or water instead of sweetened juices, squash and fizzy drinks.

○ Cut down on cakes, biscuits, sweets and chocolate as much as you can. There are lots of other things you can use for snacks:

> **Snacks**
> Fresh fruit
> raw vegetables like carrots
> pitta bread (plain, or filled with something like mashed banana)
> natural yogurt with fresh fruit
> unsweetened breakfast cereals (with milk, or dry)
> bread, with low-fat spread or a scraping of butter
> unsweetened biscuits
> popping corn, perhaps with a little grated cheese.

○ Cut down the amount of sugar in recipes. A lot of dishes are just as tasty, and often tastier, with far less sugar in them.

○ Choose breakfast cereals which are not coated in sugar or honey – they're usually cheaper. Don't sprinkle extra sugar on top.

○ Read labels on tins and packets so you will know when sugar has been added. It may be labelled as glucose, sucrose, dextrose, fructose, maltose, syrup, etc. You can buy fruit tinned in natural juices rather than in syrup. Some tins and packets are now labelled as 'low in sugar' or 'without added sugar' – but check this claim against the details on the label.

○ Aim to eat sugary things no more than three times a day at the most. One way to do this is to keep sweets, biscuits, squash and fizzy drinks for mealtimes only. It is generally best to eat sugary things along with other foods rather than alone as a snack.

(See page 50 for information about sugar and children's teeth.)

Starch and fibre

Starchy foods – bread, chappattis, breakfast cereals, rice, pasta and pulses (peas, beans of all kinds and lentils) and potatoes – are important in the diet as they are filling without having too many calories. They are also good sources of other nutrients. Eat them as replacements for fatty and sugary foods. Most starchy foods also contain fibre which helps prevent constipation. The wholegrain varieties (e.g. brown rice, wholemeal pasta) are especially rich in fibre. There is some fibre in fruit and vegetables, and these are also important for vitamins and minerals. Two easy foods that lots of children like – baked beans and frozen peas – are both good sources of fibre. Frozen peas eaten frozen make a good treat for older children – better than biscuits or sweets. Try potatoes in their skins. Just scrub them, then boil or bake. This saves time anyway.

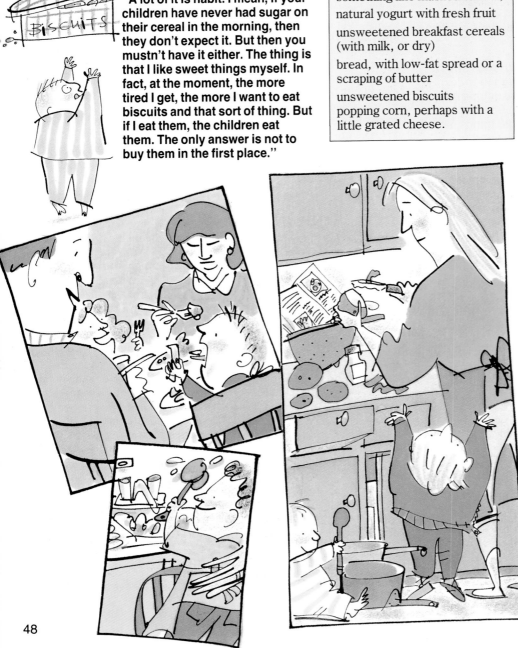

Pulses, like dried beans and lentils, are high in fibre and, because they contain protein, make a good, cheap alternative to meat. Use them more: a lot of children like them and may even prefer them to meat. Take care with cooking. Lentils don't need soaking. For other dried beans, soak for at least five hours. Soaking overnight is easiest. Then boil in fresh water for as long as needed. You must boil them for at least ten minutes to make them safe to eat. You may want to use a pressure cooker.

Get the fibre in your diet from the foods listed here. Do not add bran to increase the fibre – it can stop important minerals from being absorbed.

Protein

Everybody, but especially children, need protein for growth. Most people think about protein as coming from only a few foods, mainly meat. But in fact, most foods contain some protein. If you eat foods like fish, peas, beans, potatoes, cheese, eggs, milk and cereals, you'll be getting plenty of protein, even without eating meat or poultry at all. So it's unlikely that either you or your family is not getting enough protein.

Unless you're vegetarian, you may feel children *ought* to eat meat. But lots of children go through a phase when they won't eat meat at all, and they still get plenty of protein from other foods. Just try to make the foods that *are* eaten as varied as you can.

Not much salt

It's possible to get all the salt the body needs from the salt that is naturally found in foods. So you really don't need to add salt to any food. For some adults, too much salt may lead to high blood pressure, and children who get the taste for salty food are likely to go on eating salt as adults. Cut down on salt as much as you can. Certainly never add salt to babies' foods.

Vitamins and minerals

If you're eating a good, varied diet, including washed fruit and vegetables or salad, you're unlikely to be short of vitamins and minerals. This is true for adults and children. So once a child is eating a variety of solid foods, there shouldn't be any need to give extra vitamins.

If you have a child who simply refuses fruit and vegetables, or if you think your child may be short of vitamins for any other reason, it's sensible to go on giving vitamin drops until the age of five (see page 10).

Iron is an important mineral for young children. Meat and dark green vegetables are rich sources. It is also found in bread, eggs, nuts, beans and lentils, and absorption from these foods will be helped by consuming fruit and vegetables at the same meal. In addition, infant formula, and many infant and breakfast cereals are fortified with iron.

Fresh food as well as processed

Most families with small children eat a fair amount of processed food because it's quick and easy. But processed food does tend to contain more of just those things you need to cut down on (sugar, fat and salt) and fewer nutrients. So make sure you eat some fresh food, and food you cook yourself. When you do eat convenience food, try to avoid ones containing a lot of sugar, fat and salt. Look at labels.

Healthy fast food
Fruit and vegetables
wholemeal bread or toast
baked beans
baked potatoes
fish fingers, and frozen fish generally (but grilled or baked rather than fried)
tinned fish
tinned tomatoes
plain yogurt
cooked eggs
wholegrain breakfast cereals (which don't after all, have to be eaten at breakfast).

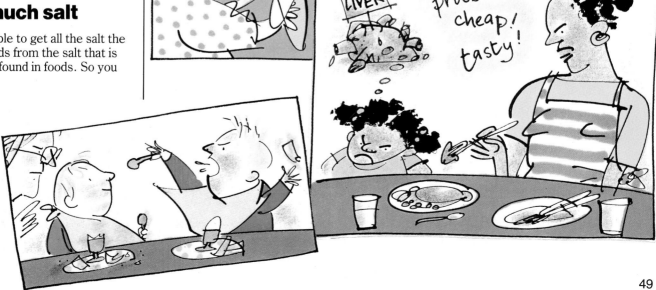

Food additives

Any additives put into food must by law be shown on the label. Many are shown by the European Community number – the 'E' number. Additives with 'E' numbers have been tested and passed as safe for use in EEC countries. Numbers without an 'E' in front are allowed in the UK but not in all EEC countries.

There is a lot of controversy at present about the use of food additives, their safety and effects – especially their effects on children. Not all additives are bad. Many are known to be safe and many are necessary, to prevent food poisoning, for example. Some are natural substances, some are synthetic. But the fact that an additive is natural doesn't make it 'safe'. Many natural additives have not been tested in the way that artificial ones have.

Vitamin D

The sunshine vitamin. Outdoor activities with some exposure of children's skin to the sun allow the skin to make vitamin D – essential for strong bones and general health.

You may be worried about the danger of skin cancer following unprotected and prolonged exposure. Take a middle road – avoid sunburn but make sure your child enjoys being out-of-doors for a while each day.

Children's teeth

To care for your child's teeth:

○ keep down the number of times each day that your child eats or drinks something sweet;

○ brush your child's teeth and gums (or help an older one to brush) thoroughly, twice each day, using a fluoride toothpaste.

Caring for teeth is very much a matter of family routine, so try to do the same for yourself as you do for your child.

Cutting down on sugar

Sugar causes tooth decay. It is not just the *amount* of sugar in sweet food and drinks that matters but, perhaps more importantly, *how often* sugary things are in the mouth. (This is why sweet drinks in a bottle, and lollipops are so bad. The teeth are bathed in sugar over quite a long time.)

○ From the time you start your baby on foods and drinks other than milk, avoid giving sweet things. Try to encourage savoury tastes. Watch for: the sugar in baby foods in tins and packets (even the savoury varieties and rusks); the huge amount of sugar in some drinks, especially fizzy drinks and the syrups which are actually advertised as

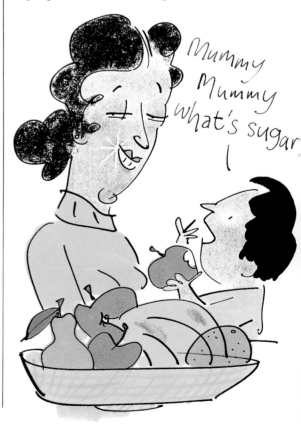

'good for babies and children' because they contain vitamins; and processed food generally, because it often contains lots of sugar. Remember to look at the labels.

○ Try not to give your child sweet foods and drinks more than three times a day. You could try keeping them for meals only. If you can cut down even more, all the better.

○ Try to find treats other than biscuits or sweets, and ask relatives and friends to do the same. Use things like stickers, badges, hair slides, crayons, small books, notebooks and colouring books, soap, bubble baths . . . These may be more expensive than one small sweet, but they all last longer, and maybe it is no bad thing if treats happen less often.

If children are given sweets or chocolate, it is actually less harmful for their teeth if they eat them all at once or in two or three goes than if they eat, say, a little every hour or so.

○ Be aware of the amount of sugar the whole family is eating. Look for ways of cutting down. (See page 48 for some suggestions.)

Toothbrushing

○ Start early, as soon as your baby's teeth start to come through. Buy a baby toothbrush and use it with a pea-sized blob of fluoride toothpaste. You don't have to use a baby toothpaste. It's much more expensive – but some children do seem happier with a milder taste. Don't worry if you don't manage to brush much at first. The important thing at the start is to get toothbrushing accepted as part of everyday routine. That's why it's important you do it too.

○ Gradually start to brush your child's teeth more thoroughly, brushing all the surfaces of all the teeth. Do it twice a day – just before bed, and whatever other time in the day fits in best. Not many children like having their teeth brushed, so you may have to work at it a bit. Try not to let it become a battle. If it becomes difficult, try games, or try brushing your own teeth at the same time then helping your child to 'finish off'.

○ Go on helping your child to brush until you are sure he or she is brushing well enough. You'll probably have to keep an eye on brushing until your child is a teenager.

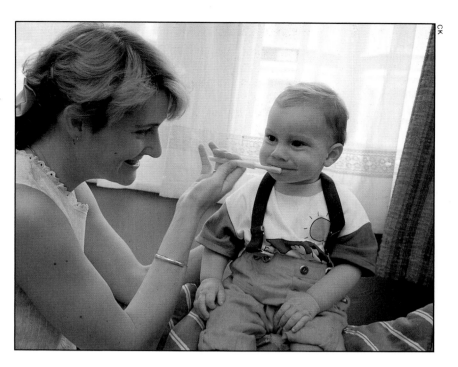

Fluoride

Fluoride is a chemical which helps prevent tooth decay. In a few areas, it is naturally present in the water supply, and in others, it is added. But if you live in an area without fluoride in the water supply, you can give your child fluoride supplements. Talk to your health visitor and/or your dentist about whether you need to give them.

Fluoride supplements come as drops (for babies) and tablets (for older children). You can buy them from the chemist.

Going to the dentist

All your child's teeth should be through by two or three years of age, so this is the latest that visits to the dentist should start. It's worthwhile taking your baby along earlier, before the teeth appear, as the dentist can give preventive advice. Take your child with you when you go to the dentist for a check-up. If your child can get to know the dentist and the surgery, it may help later.

If you have trouble finding a dentist, ask at your local clinic. There may be a children's dental service there.

Dental treatment is free for children under the age of 18.

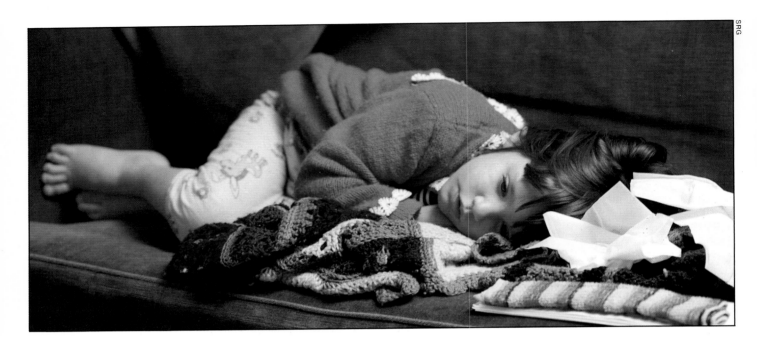

Illness

Knowing when your child is ill

Sometimes there's no doubt. But often it is difficult to tell whether a child is ill. Children can be listless, hot and miserable one minute, running around quite happily the next.

Remember that:

○ what you should watch for is some sign of illness (like vomiting, or a temperature) *plus* behaviour that's unusual for your child (like a lot of crying, being very irritable, or refusing food).

○ possible signs of illness are always more worrying in a baby or very small child. See page 21 for when to consult the doctor about your baby.

For older children, if you are uncertain whether or not to see the doctor, you might want to carry on normally for a while and see whether the signs of illness or pain continue. It might be best not to let your child see you're watching. Most can put on an act, especially if they see you're worried.

Above all, trust your feelings. You know better than anyone what your child is like day to day, so you'll know what's unusual or worrying. If you are worried, contact your doctor.

Using your doctor

Your health visitor and/or clinic doctor can give you advice and help you decide whether your child is really unwell or not. But it is only your family doctor (your GP) who can treat your child and prescribe medicines. If you think your child is ill, it's best to see your family doctor.

If you are unsure whether to go to the surgery or ask for a home visit, phone and talk to the receptionist or to your doctor. Explain how your child is and what's worrying you. Often it doesn't do a child (or anyone else) any harm to be taken to the surgery, and you are likely to get attention more quickly this way. But explain if it's difficult for you to get there. Wrapping a sick child up and going by car is one thing; going on the bus might be impossible.

If you are seriously worried and/or know your child needs urgent attention, phone your doctor at any time of the day or night. There may be a different number for when the surgery is closed. See inside back cover for what to do in an emergency.

Using medicines

You may want to use medicines as little as possible. That's usually wise, although sometimes medicine *is* the right and best answer. If you are offered a prescription but would rather not give your child medicine, talk with your doctor about whether it is really needed, why, how it will help, and whether there are any alternatives.

○ Make sure you understand how much and

how often to give a medicine. Write it down if need be. If in doubt, check with your chemist or doctor.

○ When a medicine is prescribed, ask about any possible side effects. Could it, for example, make your child sleepy or irritable?

○ Always finish a course of medicine. A course of antibiotics, for example, usually lasts at least five days. This is to make sure all the bacteria are killed off. Your child may seem better after two or three days, but the illness is more likely to return if you don't finish all the medicine.

○ If you think your child is reacting badly to a medicine (for example, with a rash or diarrhoea), stop giving it and tell your doctor. Keep a note of the medicine so you can make sure you don't get it another time.

○ If you buy medicines at the chemist, always say it is for a young child. Give your child's age. Some medicines are for adults only. Always follow the instructions on the label.

> **Aspirin** should not be given to children under twelve. It has now been linked with a rare but dangerous illness. Use **paracetamol** instead, making sure you have got the right strength for your child. Read the label and/or check with your chemist.

○ Look for the date stamp. Don't use out-of-date medicines. Flush them down the lavatory.

○ Only give your child medicine given by your doctor or chemist. Never use medicines prescribed for anyone else.

○ Keep all medicines out of children's reach, locked away if possible.

○ Medicines in liquid form often contain large amounts of sugar which may contribute to tooth decay. If your child has to take liquid medicine, especially over a long period of time, ask for a sugar-free one.

○ Small doses of liquid medicines may need to be given using a Liquid Medicine Measure. Always read the manufacturer's instructions supplied with the measure and always give the exact dose stated on the medicine bottle.

○ Brush your child's teeth after giving medicine.

Looking after a sick child

○ Look after your child yourself if you can. If you can't be at home (and for working parents it's sometimes impossible), try to

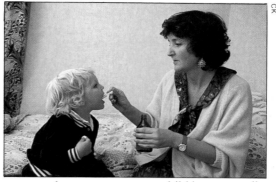

arrange for someone your child knows well to do the caring.

○ It doesn't matter if your child doesn't want to stay in bed. Being with you, maybe tucked up in an armchair or on a sofa, might be less lonely. Children are usually sensible about being ill and if they say they're well enough to be out of bed, they very likely are.

○ Keep the room warm (not hot) and airy.

○ See page 55 for what to do if your child has a temperature.

○ Give plenty to drink. For the first day or so, don't bother about food unless it's wanted. After that, try to find ways of making a bit of food tempting.

○ Lay on lots of entertainment. Distraction does help. Try to give time for games, stories, company and comforting.

○ Sick children are often easily tired and need lots of rest. Encourage your child to doze off when he or she needs to, perhaps with a story, read by you or on a tape.

Looking after a sick child, even for a couple of days, is exhausting. Make things as easy for yourself as you can, get rest and sleep when you can, and try to get somebody else to take over every now and then to give you a break.

When you're ill yourself

"Mothers can't be ill. You just have to soldier on. But it means it takes you longer to get over something."

When you're ill yourself, even just with a bout of flu, life can become very difficult. A lot of parents have to ignore their own illnesses. But there does come a point when it is wrong to soldier on. If you can only get some rest, get yourself to the doctor, look after yourself (or better still, be looked after) for a bit, you may get better again more quickly. Try to get help so you can stay in bed if you need to. If you are really in difficulty, explain your situation to your health visitor.

Common complaints

Colds

○ The reason why children get so many colds is that there are hundreds of different cold viruses. Young children are meeting each one of them for the first time. Gradually they build up some immunity and get fewer colds.

○ Colds are caused by viruses not bacteria, so antibiotics don't help.

○ Sometimes babies who are snuffly can't breathe easily when feeding or asleep. Your doctor may prescribe nose drops which can help, or you could try gently tickling your baby's nostrils with some cotton wool; a sneeze might help to clear the nose.

○ A menthol rub, or capsules containing a decongestant liquid (which you can put onto clothes, or a cloth) may help your child breathe more freely, especially at night. You can buy them from chemists. You can also buy vapourisers, which can be helpful but are expensive.

Colic

See page 17.

Constipation

See page 20 (babies) and page 44.

Coughs

○ Most coughs, like colds, are caused by a virus, so antibiotics don't usually help. But if the cough is bad and won't go away, see your doctor. If your child has a chest infection, then an antibiotic may be needed – although it won't soothe or stop the cough straightaway. Sometimes a bad cough, especially one with a wheeze, is a sign of asthma. Your doctor can check this and give treatment.

○ A teaspoon of honey in squeezed orange or lemon juice and warm water is just as soothing as cough mixture. Whatever the manufacturers may tell you, most cough mixtures are a waste of money. In fact, coughing serves a purpose. When there is phlegm on the chest, or mucus from the nose runs down the back of the throat, coughing clears it away. You'll probably want to soothe a cough, but there's no need to try to stop it.

○ A steamy atmosphere may help if the cough is 'croupy'. You could take your baby into the bathroom with you while you have a steamy bath, or have older children playing in the bathroom. But be careful. Very hot water, even if it isn't boiling, can scald.

Croup causes the back of the throat to swell, making breathing difficult. It brings hoarse coughing, and noisy breaths-in. See your doctor if you think your child has croup. If it is affecting breathing it needs to be treated urgently.

Diarrhoea

○ Young babies' stools are naturally runny and yellow or orange coloured. But if you notice anything unusual about your baby's stools and there are other signs of illness too, see your doctor.

> Young babies who get diarrhoea can lose a lot of fluid, especially if they are being sick as well, if the weather is hot, or they have a fever. This can be dangerous. You need to see your doctor as soon as possible. In the meantime, give your baby plenty of fluid. Carry on breast feeding, feeding more often if possible. Or, if you are bottle feeding, stop giving formula milk and give boiled cooled water, adding half a teaspoon of sugar and a pinch of salt to every 8 fluid ounces of water.

○ In older children, diarrhoea isn't usually worrying. Give plenty of clear drinks to keep fluids up, but only give food if it's wanted. If the diarrhoea goes on for longer than two or three days, see your doctor.

Ear infections

○ These are common in babies and small children. They often follow a cold and sometimes cause a bit of a temperature. Your child may pull or rub at an ear, but babies can't always tell where pain is coming from and may just cry and seem unwell and uncomfortable.

○ If you suspect an ear infection, take your child to the doctor. It's important, so go as soon as you can. Ear infections can cause hearing problems and need to be dealt with. Paracetamol may help lessen pain in the meantime.

Flu-like illnesses

○ Infections caused by one sort of virus or another are easily passed around, especially once children start to mix together. Most children get flu-like illnesses every now and then. Your child will probably be just mildly unwell and generally miserable. There may be a cold, a slight temperature, a headache, aching muscles and joints, a sore throat, a cough.

○ Your child may want to stay in bed or be tucked up in an armchair, or may want to be up and about. Give rest, plenty of cool drinks, and paracetamol to bring a temperature down and ease aching and discomfort. There is no need to see your doctor unless you become worried.

Head lice

○ Lots of children get head lice. It makes no difference whether their hair is clean or dirty. They catch them just by coming into contact with someone who is infected. When heads touch, the lice simple walk from one head to the other.

○ An itchy scalp is often the first sign that a child has head lice. But by this time, the lice have probably been in the hair for several weeks. So check your child's hair regularly – say, every time it's washed. You're looking for tiny white/grey eggs (or nits) which are laid close to the scalp. Unlike dandruff, they're firmly attached to the hair and can't be shaken off.

○ If you do find your child has head lice, get treatment straightaway. Ask your health visitor, clinic, doctor or chemist. Treatment is usually a lotion which kills the lice and eggs. Follow the instructions carefully. Treat the whole family as lice spread very easily.

○ The lotion kills the lice and nits but the nits don't wash off. You'll still be able to see some in the hair. It doesn't mean your child is still infected. If you want to get rid of the dead nits, you can use a special nit comb. You can buy one at the chemist.

○ After treatment, there's no need to keep your child off nursery or school.

○ Check that no-one else is infected, not just in the family but also your child's friends.

○ Brush and comb hair often. It helps prevent head lice taking hold.

Nappy rash
See page 20.

Sore throat

○ Many sore throats are caused by virus illnesses like colds or flu. The throat may be dry, sore and itchy for a day or so before the cold starts.

○ Sometimes a sore throat is caused by tonsillitis. Your child may find it hard to swallow, have a high temperature, and swollen glands at the front of the neck, high up under the jaw.

○ If your child has a sore throat and a high temperature, or is generally unwell, check with your doctor. If the sore throat is caused by a virus, antibiotics won't be needed. But if the cause is tonsillitis, antibiotics usually help.

Teething
See page 27.

Temperatures

○ For babies, always contact your doctor if there are other signs of illness along with a raised temperature and/or if your baby's temperature is over 38.5°C/101°F. (If you think your baby is ill, with or without a raised temperature, it's best to see your doctor anyway.)

○ In older children, a little fever isn't usually a worry. But contact your doctor if your child seems unusually ill, or if the temperature is high and doesn't come down. Otherwise, give as much to drink as your child wants. Cold, clear drinks are best. Even if your child's not thirsty, try to get him or her to drink a little and often, to keep fluids up. Don't bother about food unless it's wanted.

○ It's important to try to bring a temperature down, not just to

To take a baby's or young child's temperature, first shake down the mercury in the thermometer. Hold your child on your knee and tuck the thermometer under his or her armpit. Hold your child's arm against his or her body. Leave the thermometer in place for three minutes. (It may help to read a story or watch television while you do this.)
By about five years old, many children will take a thermometer under their tongue in the normal way.
   Normal body temperature, taken under the tongue, is about 37°C/98.4°F, but may vary a bit. Taken under the arm, normal temperature is slightly lower – about 36.4°C/97.4°F.
   Strip-type thermometers which you hold on your child's forehead are not an accurate way of taking temperatures. They show the skin, not the body temperature.

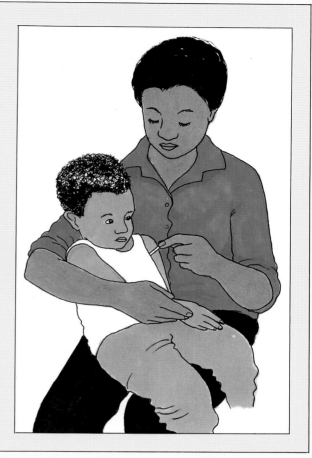

make your child more comfortable, but also because a continuing high temperature can be very unpleasant and, in a small child, occasionally brings on a fit or convulsion. So don't wrap your child up. Take off a layer of clothing. Let older children wear light clothes, or lie naked under a sheet. Sponging your child's body, arms and legs with tepid water can also help. Don't dry the skin. As the water evaporates, it takes heat out of the body. Give cool drinks. Paracetamol will also help to lower the temperature.

Threadworms

○ Lots of children get threadworms. You will see them in your child's stools, looking like tiny white threads. Your child may have an itchy bottom and may scratch it a lot, especially at night.

○ If you think your child has worms, see your doctor, or ask your chemist for treatment. Everybody in the family has to be treated because the threadworm eggs spread very easily.

○ To prevent the infection spreading, make sure that everybody in the family washes their hands well and scrubs their nails before every meal and after going to the toilet.

Vomiting

○ Almost all babies sick up a bit of milk, some a lot, without distress. But if your baby is vomiting often or violently and/or there are other signs of illness, contact your doctor straight away. Babies can lose a dangerous amount of fluid if they are sick often, especially if they have diarrhoea as well. See the boxed information under 'Diarrhoea' for how to keep your baby's fluids up.

○ Older children can be sick once or twice, without any bother, and be well again very quickly afterwards, or after a night's sleep. If the vomiting goes on, and/or there are other signs of illness, contact your doctor.

○ Give plenty to drink – clear drinks rather than milk. Don't bother about food unless it's wanted.

Infectious illnesses

Note: Rashes look different on different people. The colours of spots can vary, and on a black skin, rashes may be less easy to see. If in doubt, check with your doctor.

Meningitis

Meningitis is caused by bacteria or viruses which infect the membranes covering the brain. It can be a serious disease, especially in babies and young children. Although early treatment often brings about a complete cure, meningitis can cause various sorts of handicap, including brain damage.

There are two main types of the disease. **Bacterial** meningitis is less common, more serious, and needs urgent treatment with antibiotics. **Viral** meningitis is more common, usually less serious and can't be helped by antibiotics. It is often difficult to tell the difference between bacterial and viral meningitis without hospital tests.

Meningitis is rare, but recent outbreaks of one of the serious bacterial types, **meningococcal meningitis**, have made it a cause for concern. There is another type of meningitis caused by a bacteria called Hib *(Haemophilus influenzae b)*. In the UK, it is the most common form of bacterial meningitis in the under four-year-olds, and most dangerous to children under one year. The germs causing this type of meningitis are found in the noses and throats of people who are perfectly well. It isn't known why some people who carry the germs develop meningitis and some do not. Children are more likely to be affected than adults because they have less natural immunity.

How to recognise it

Meningitis can develop very rapidly. Babies may refuse foods, have a staring expression, or a rigid body. They may be fretful, make a shrill or moaning cry, especially when handled. They may be difficult to wake up. In young children it usually begins with a high fever, headache and vomiting. Your child may be unusually irritable. It is very important to get a doctor's advice at the earliest possible stage of the illness. Later, other signs may develop – such as pain and stiffness in the back of the neck, and dislike of light. These symptoms may not all appear at the same time, *or at all*.

What to do

If you are worried about your child, call your doctor straight away to get advice. It is important to recognise meningitis early. The earlier treatment is started, the better the chance of complete recovery. If your child becomes confused, limp or floppy, or possibly unconscious, and if your doctor is not available, take your child straight to the accident and emergency department of the nearest hospital with a children's unit.

Hib, measles, mumps, rubella and whooping cough can all be prevented by immunisation. See pages 59-61 for information.

HEPATITIS B
See page 58.

	Incubation period (the time between catching an illness and becoming unwell)	Infectious period (when your child can give the illness to someone else)
Chickenpox	14-16 days.	From the day before the rash appears until the spots are dry.
Measles	7-12 days.	From a few days before the rash appears until 5 days after it goes.
Mumps	14-21 days.	From a few days before becoming unwell until swelling goes down. Maybe 10 days in all.
Rubella (German measles)	14-21 days.	From a few days before illness starts until a week after the rash first appears.
Whooping cough	7-14 days.	From the first signs of illness until about 6 weeks after coughing first started, unless an antibiotic is given.

How to recognise it	What to do
Begins with feeling unwell, a rash and maybe a slight temperature. Spots are red and become fluid-filled blisters within a day or so. Come first on the chest and back, then spread. The spots eventually dry into scabs, which drop off. Unless spots are badly infected, they don't usually leave a scar.	No need to see the doctor unless you are unsure whether it's chickenpox or your child is very unwell and/or distressed. Give plenty to drink. Paracetamol will help bring down a temperature. Baths, loose comfortable clothes and calamine lotion can all ease the itchiness.
Begins like a bad cold and cough. Child becomes gradually more unwell, with a temperature. Rash appears after 3rd or 4th day. Spots are red and slightly raised; may be blotchy. Rash is not itchy. Child becomes very unwell, with cough and high temperature. Illness usually lasts about a week.	See your doctor. Give rest, and plenty to drink. Warm drinks will ease the cough. Paracetamol will ease discomfort and lower the temperature. Vaseline around the lips protects the skin. Wash crustiness from eyelids with warm water. See pages 59-61 for information about immunisation against measles.
At first, child may be mildly unwell with a bit of fever. May complain of pain around the ear or feel uncomfortable when chewing. Swelling then starts, under the jaw up by the ear. Swelling often starts on one side, followed (though not always) by the other. Face is back to normal size in about a week. (It is rare for mumps to affect boys testes. This happens rather more often in adult men with mumps. For both boys and men, the risk of any permanent damage to the testes is very low.)	Child may not feel especially ill and may not want to be in bed. Paracetamol will ease pain in the swollen glands. Give plenty to drink, but not fruit juices. They make the saliva flow, which can hurt. No need to see the doctor unless your child has stomach-ache and is being sick. See pages 59-61 for information about immunisation against mumps.
Can be difficult to diagnose with certainty. Starts like a mild cold. Rash appears in a day or two, first on the face, then spreading. Spots are flat. On a light skin, they are pale pink. Glands in the back of the neck may be swollen. Child doesn't usually feel unwell. Give plenty to drink.	Keep your child away from anybody you know who is pregnant (or trying to become so). If your child was with anyone pregnant before you knew about the illness, let them know. If a pregnant woman catches German measles, there is a risk of damage to her baby. Any pregnant woman who has had contact with German measles should see her doctor. The doctor can check whether or not she is immune, and if not, whether there is any sign of her developing the illness. See pages 59-61 for information about immunisation against rubella.
Begins like a cold and cough. The cough gradually gets worse. After about 2 weeks, coughing bouts start. These are exhausting and make it difficult to breathe. Sometimes, but not always, there's a whooping noise as the child draws in breath after coughing. It takes some weeks before the coughing fits start to die down.	If your child has a cough that gets worse rather than better and starts to have longer fits of coughing more and more often, see your doctor. It's important for the sake of other children to know whether or not it's whooping cough. Talk to your doctor about how best to look after your child. See pages 59-61 for information about immunisation against whooping cough.

Hepatitis B

Hepatitis means inflammation of the liver. This can be caused by hepatitis B which can be transmitted from an infected mum to her baby during pregnancy or at birth. This baby will probably not be ill, but will usually become a carrier of the virus. This can cause liver disease later in life. However, this is now preventable.

Nowadays, mothers-to-be are often screened for the virus using a simple blood test. Babies born to infected mothers are then started very soon after birth on a three-dose course of hepatitis B vaccine. This prevents them from becoming infected.

If you would like to know more about hepatitis B virus or hepatitis B immunisation, your health visitor or GP will be happy to talk to you.

(It is OK for an infected mum to breast feed, provided the baby has had the immunisation.)

Children in hospital

Hospitals are strange, frightening places for children. Being ill or in pain is frightening too. There's no parent who isn't anxious to do all they can to help their child through.

○ Prepare your child as best you can. You could play 'doctors and nurses' or 'operations' with teddies and dolls and read story books about being in hospital. It's worth doing this even if you don't know your child is going into hospital. Quite a high number of under-five year olds do have to go into hospital at some stage, and many go in as emergencies.

○ It's extremely important for you to be with your child in hospital as much as possible and, with young children especially, to sleep there. Do all you can to arrange this. Most hospitals are helpful, but at some you do have to push.

○ Talk to hospital staff beforehand and be clear about arrangements, what will happen, and so on. You may then be able to explain at least a part of it to your child.

○ Even quite young children need to know about what is happening to them, so explaining as much as possible is important.

What children imagine is often worse than reality. Be truthful, too. Don't, for example, say something won't hurt when it will.

○ Talk with hospital staff about anything that will be important for your child. You may need to explain cultural differences. Staff should know, for example, if hospital food is going to seem very strange to your child. Try to discuss ways of getting over problems like this.

Also tell staff about any special words your child uses (such as for needing to go to the lavatory), any special ways of comforting, and so on.

○ Make sure something like a favourite teddy bear or comforter goes into hospital with your child.

○ Be prepared for your child to be upset by the experience, and maybe to show it in one way or another for some time afterwards. Reassure as much as you can.

You can get a lot of helpful information and advice on how best to cope when your child is in hospital from the National Association for the Welfare of Children in Hospital (NAWCH – address on page 94).

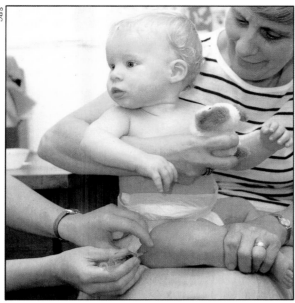

SRG

Immunisation – the safest way to protect your child

Hib, whooping cough, diphtheria, tetanus, polio, tuberculosis, measles, mumps and rubella (German measles). These diseases are more serious than people think – and sometimes they are fatal.

Immunisation protects your child. It's quick, simple and safe.

The more children who are immunised, the rarer the diseases become. So immunisation protects not only your child but young babies, other children and adults as well.

The purpose of this section is to help you to understand the benefits of immunisation.

Why immunise?

These children's diseases are serious . . .

Hib causes a range of diseases: one type of meningitis, epiglottitis (which can cause a blocked windpipe), infections of the bones and joints, blood poisoning and pneumonia. In the UK, it has been responsible for 65 deaths each year and 150 children are left with permanent brain damage.

Whooping cough is very infectious and can cause long, distressing bouts of coughing and choking. These bouts are exhausting and frightening, and can happen up to 50 times a day. The illness itself usually lasts about three to four weeks. The coughing may go on for much longer.

Whooping cough can cause convulsions (fits), ear infections, pneumonia, bronchitis, collapsed lungs and sometimes brain damage.

Diphtheria is another serious and, sometimes, fatal illness. It begins with a simple sore throat, but quickly develops into a serious illness which can last for weeks. It blocks the nose or throat making it difficult, sometimes nearly impossible, for the child to breathe. Diphtheria is now very rare in Britain because so many children are immunised against it. But it is still a disease that can kill.

Tetanus is caused by germs from soil, dirt or dust getting into an open wound (especially a deep 'puncture' wound) or burn. It attacks the nervous system causing painful muscle spasms. Because of immunisation it's now quite rare, but there is still a real chance of getting it and it can be fatal.

Polio no longer exists in this country because of widespread immunisation, but could still recur. It attacks the nervous system causing muscle paralysis in any part of the body. When it affects the breathing muscles a child may have to be helped to breathe artificially and even then may die. If it affects the legs, they become weak or even paralysed – sometimes permanently.

Because many families travel abroad, there is a risk of coming into contact with polio, even though it does not occur in this country.

Care is needed in handling the nappies of children who have just received the polio immunisation and for 30 days after each dose. As always, wash your hands after changing baby's nappy.

Measles is very common and highly infectious. Beginning like a bad cold, it develops into a fever and a rash. The child with measles always feels very miserable and may be very unwell with a bad cough and a high temperature.

Measles is much more serious than most people think. In fact, of all childhood infections, it is the one most likely to cause encephalitis (inflammation of the brain), sometimes resulting in brain damage. It can also cause convulsions and ear infections; and bronchitis and pneumonia, which can lead to long-term lung troubles. Measles can kill.

Mumps is usually a mild illness, but it can have serious complications. It is the most common cause of viral meningitis among the under 15s and can cause permanent deafness. *Mumps is equally dangerous for boys and girls.*

Rubella (German measles) is a mild disease but if a pregnant woman who is not immune catches it, then her unborn baby can be damaged. The risk is especially high if it is caught in the first four months of pregnancy. The baby may then be born deaf, blind and with heart and brain damage.

The most likely way for a mother to catch rubella is through contact with a small child (boy or girl) who has it. So it's important for all children to be immunised.

The vaccines and how to protect your child

The vaccines which immunise against diphtheria, whooping cough and tetanus are combined into one triple vaccine called DTP – Diphtheria, Tetanus and Pertussis (the medical name for whooping cough). It is given as three injections during your child's first year: at 2 months, 3 months, and 4 months. All three are necessary for maximum immunity.

Hib vaccine is given at 2, 3 and 4 months – at the same time as DTP injections. After the course of injections, no booster dose is necessary.

Polio vaccine is given as drops by mouth. It is given in three doses at the same time as the triple (DTP) vaccine.

The vaccines which immunise against measles, mumps and rubella are also combined into one injection. This combined vaccine is known as MMR. The best time to have it is between 12 and 15 months, but it can be given at any later age. Even if you think your child has already had one of these diseases, your child should still have the MMR vaccine.

Booster immunisations against diphtheria, tetanus and polio are given at the time children enter school.

The timetable

Although babies have some natural immunity, whether bottle or breast fed, it only lasts a short time. And diseases like whooping cough are most dangerous in the very youngest children. In fact, there are more deaths in the under-ones from this disease than all the other age groups combined. So early protection is important.

The timetable also means that the immunisations can be completed while your child is visiting the clinic/doctor regularly.

And before you go back to work. It's a timetable that everyone can remember, the same across the country. More information is contained in the leaflet, *Guide to childhood immunisations,* available from your health visitor or GP.

Immunisation timetable

At 2 months		
Hib		one injection
Diphtheria Tetanus Whooping cough	}	DTP one injection
Polio		by mouth
At 3 months		
Hib		one injection
Diphtheria Tetanus Whooping cough	}	DTP one injection
Polio		by mouth
At 4 months		
Hib		one injection
Diphtheria Tetanus Whooping cough	}	DTP one injection
Polio		by mouth
At 12-18 months	**(usually before 15 months)**	
Measles Mumps Rubella	}	MMR one injection
3-5 years	**(around school entry)**	
Diphtheria Tetanus	}	booster injections
Polio		booster by mouth

Immunisation against **tuberculosis** is also offered to children who, for whatever reasons, are at greater risk of catching this disease. This immunisation is given shortly after birth.

If your child has missed any of these immunisations, or started them late, don't worry. Your doctor will tell you how to fit them in so that your child is fully protected.

Worries about reactions and side effects

After any of these immunisations, children may feel a bit unwell for a while or be irritable or even have a temperature. Contact the doctor if you are worried, and especially if your child has a temperature, becomes jittery or screams. If your baby is aged between two and three months, your doctor should advise you that a 2½ml dose of baby paracetamol will help bring down any temperature. If your baby is older, the dose can be 2½ml or 5ml. If you are not sure which dose to give, your doctor or pharmacist will advise you. You can get a special oral syringe from the pharmacist for measuring the right amount.

Sometimes the skin becomes red, sore or swollen around the place where the injection was given, or a small lump appears and may take a few weeks to disappear. *Don't worry, this is perfectly normal.* If your child is due to have his or her next triple (DTP) vaccine, there's no need to delay the injections.

Triple immunisation

Side effects from the triple vaccine (DTP) are almost always mild. Your baby may become fretful and slightly feverish within 24 hours of the injection.

Very rarely, a child may have a convulsion as a result of fever after the immunisation. If this happens, the child usually recovers quickly with no lasting effects. The chances of more serious side effects are very remote indeed.

The whooping cough part of the triple vaccine is the one which some parents worry about most. Many people know how dangerous the disease can be, especially among the very youngest children, but remain unsure about whooping cough immunisation because of fears in the past about its safety. In fact, millions of children have been immunised against whooping cough without any harm whatsoever, and these fears are unnecessary.

After a very careful British study, the largest in the world, we have learned that if the vaccine did cause damage, such damage, if it occurs at all, is so rare that we can't even accurately measure it.

We believe you can be confident that the whooping cough vaccine is safe. You can protect your child from dangerous illness with a safe vaccine.

Hib immunisation

About one child in ten may develop a small red swelling about the size of an old 10 pence piece after the Hib immunisation. This usually appears within 3 to 4 hours and disappears within 48 hours. (The reaction, if any, will be less with each dose). Giving your baby the Hib immunisation at the same time as the DTP does not cause any greater reaction or side effects.

MMR immunisation

Most children are perfectly well after having the MMR (Measles, Mumps and Rubella) vaccine. However, it is quite common for children to develop a mild fever and a rash, a week to ten days later, which should only last for two to three days. A few children get swollen faces or a mild form of mumps about three weeks after MMR. Any swelling will gradually go down. *None of these reactions are infectious.*

Serious reactions to the MMR vaccine, like a convulsion with fever or encephalitis (inflammation of the brain), are extremely rare and far more likely to happen as a result of having the diseases themselves. The MMR vaccine has been used safely in other countries, particularly the United States, where millions of children have received it for many years.

Worried about complications?

The risk of harmful complications from any of these vaccines is extremely small indeed. The risks of harmful effects from the diseases themselves are much more serious.

Some parents worry about possible harmful effects from immunisations but vaccines have been given to many millions of children without any problems, and to enormous benefit.

If your child is unwell on the day and has a fever, then discuss this with your doctor or health visitor. There are very few genuine reasons why immunisations should not be done, but you might hear all sorts of stories about immunisations that actually are not true. Get the best advice from your GP, doctor or health visitor.

Does immunisation guarantee my child will be protected?

Almost all children get long-lasting and effective protection from these diseases. Very rarely, the vaccine may not give complete protection and then your child could catch the disease. The Hib immunisation **only** protects against Hib infection. It does not protect against other forms of meningitis (viral, meningococcal, or pneumococcal).

Safety

● Accidents are the commonest cause of death among children aged between one and five.

● Every year, about half a million children under five go to hospital because of an accident in the home. That is one in every six under-five year olds.

There is bound to be a limit to what you can do to protect your child from accidents. You certainly *can* do a lot to make your own home safe, although even here you may be limited by the kind of place you live in. You probably *can't* do much about what's outside your front door – roads, playgrounds, stairs and walkways, for example. Even so, parents have sometimes managed to get things changed by together putting pressure on their local council.

Simply do all that you can to keep your child safe. And don't ever rely on your child's good behaviour or common sense. Gradually you'll be able to teach your child about safety, and explain dangers. But *you can't depend* on your child remembering what you've said.

GETTING ADVICE

You can get more information and advice on how to prevent accidents from:

Your health visitor

A home safety officer
A road safety officer
(Phone your local authority – in the phone book under your authority's name.)

A fire prevention officer
(Contact your local fire brigade.)

RoSPA (The Royal Society for the Prevention of Accidents – address on page 95). RoSPA produce helpful publications, for children as well as for parents.

Safety checklist

Use this list to check what you can do to prevent accidents. It is impossible to list all dangers, but thinking about some should start you thinking about others.

Danger – of choking and suffocation

○ Keep small objects away from babies and small children who might put them in their mouths.

○ Watch out for ribbons and strings that might, either in play or by accident, get wound round a child's neck.

○ Don't give children under seven peanuts. They often cause choking.

○ Keep all polythene bags out of children's reach.

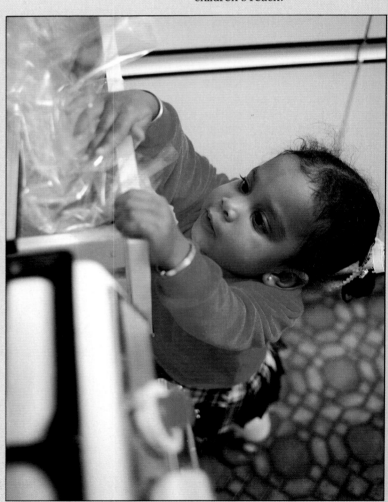

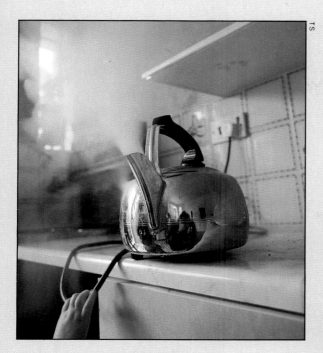

Danger – of burns and scalds

○ Keep everything hot out of children's reach. Watch for dangling flexes from irons and kettles that a child might pull on. You can get coiled kettle flex.

○ Use a fire guard, fixed to the wall, round any kind of open fire (coal, gas or electric) or a hot stove.

○ Turn pan handles away from the front edge of a cooker. Fit a cooker safety guard. Or use a safety gate across the kitchen doorway, a playpen or even the cot to keep your child safe while you cook. A flat work surface on either side of a cooker will prevent your child reaching pan handles at the side of the cooker.

○ Don't drink anything hot with your child on your lap. Keep your child away when you're carrying hot drinks, and put mugs and cups, coffee jugs and teapots out of reach. Watch for tablecloths: pulling at the edges can bring a hot drink or teapot down on a child.

○ Run some cold water in the bath first and always test the temperature before your child gets in. Be especially careful once your child is big enough to get into the bath without help. Never leave your child alone in the bath: the taps are tempting to play with. And a baby can drown in even a small amount of water.

Danger – of falls

○ Put babies in bouncing chairs on the floor, not a table or worktop.

○ For babies who are crawling and unsteady toddlers, use a properly fixed stair gate, preferably at both top and bottom of stairs.

○ Baby walkers can be dangerous. Watch out for the danger of it tipping over on steps or down stairs, or getting caught against a radiator or fire.

○ Check rails round landings and balconies. Could your child fall through, crawl under, climb over? Horizontal railings are especially dangerous.

○ Make sure upstairs windows won't open wide enough for a child to fall out. Fit safety catches if needed.

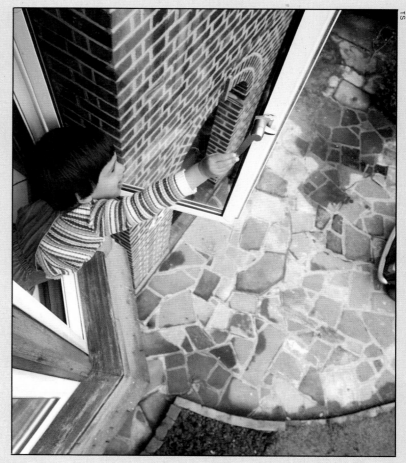

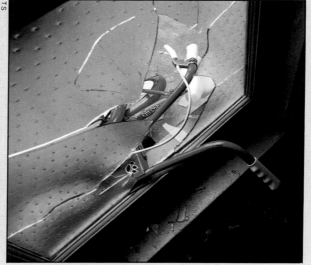

Danger – of cuts

○ Low-level glass in doors and windows is dangerous, especially once your child is on the move. Board it up, fit safety film, or even better, safety glass.

○ Keep all sharp things away from children.

○ Don't let children walk around holding anything made of glass, or with anything like a pencil or lollipop stick in their mouths.

Danger – of poisoning

○ Lock medicines away. Don't keep even the odd bottle out. Ask the chemist to put your medicines in child-resistant containers.

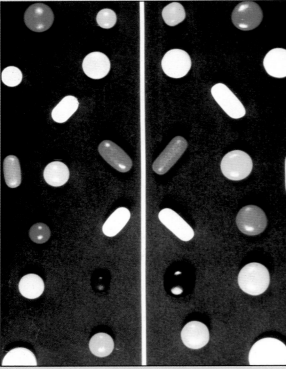

On the left are drugs, on the right are sweets.

○ Watch your child when you're in other people's houses. Watch for dangers like tablets in drawers, handbags etc.

○ Keep household and garden chemicals, and also alcohol, in a safe place, high up, or locked away. Some chemicals are sold with child-resistant caps. Make sure you replace the cap properly after use.

○ Don't put dangerous liquids in any bottle or jar that could make them look like a drink.

○ Don't let your child pick and eat any plants, fungi, berries or seeds.

○ If you use surma on your child's eyes, make sure you use one of the safe, lead-free brands. Talk to your chemist. Some surma can be dangerous.

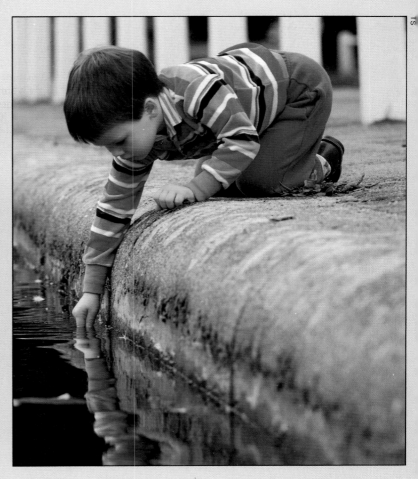

Danger – of drowning

○ Never leave a baby or young child alone in the bath, not for a moment. If the phone or doorbell rings, take your child with you, or let it ring.

○ Always watch and stay near children playing in or near water – ponds, paddling pools, the sea. If you have a garden pond, cover it up, fence it off, or get rid of it altogether. Teach your child to swim as soon as possible.

Danger – from electricity

○ Cover electric sockets with safety covers when not in use. Or put heavy furniture in front.

○ Repair worn flexes.

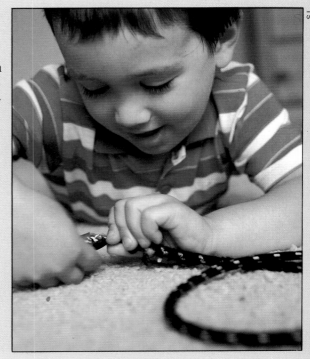

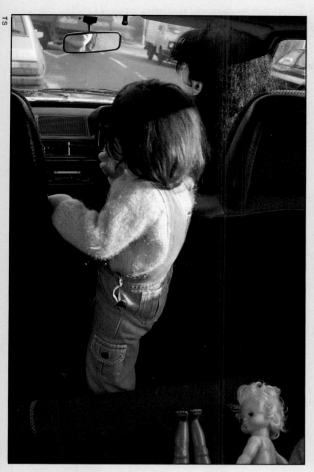

Danger — in cars

○ The *only* safe way for anybody, adult or child, to travel in a car is properly restrained. Use proper restraints for your child from the start. Older children sometimes make a fuss, but if you make it a habit that is *never* broken, your child will eventually accept that being in a car means being strapped in.

○ It is not only extremely dangerous but also illegal to hold a baby in your arms in the front seat of a car, or to let a young child travel in the front seat without a restraint. It is very dangerous to hold a baby or child on your lap anywhere in a car.

○ Babies should travel –
either in a special baby seat, facing backwards and strapped onto the back or front seat by the existing adult seat belt;
or in a carrycot fastened to the back seat with a special safety harness.

A special baby seat is safest.

In a growing number of areas there are loan schemes for baby safety seats. Through these schemes, you can get the seats more cheaply. Some schemes are run by local maternity hospitals. Or ask your midwife, health visitor or road safety officer.

○ Older children should travel on the back seat, strapped into a child safety seat or, later, on a booster cushion and strapped in with a child's safety harness or adult seat belt. Make sure any harness or seat belt fits snugly.

If you are in somebody else's car and there is no child safety seat or harness, make your child use an adult seat belt, ideally in the back, and with a special booster cushion. An adult seat belt is better than no restraint at all. Standing on the back seat, or in the gap between the two front seats, is *very* dangerous.

○ Don't let children travel in the rear luggage compartment of hatchback or estate cars, unless specially adapted by the manufacturer with seats and belts.

○ By law, anyone travelling in the rear seat of a car, must use an *appropriate restraint* if one is fitted.

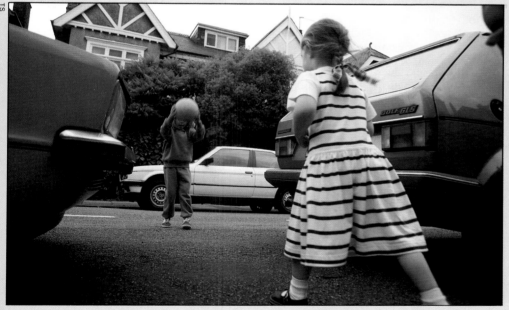

Danger — on the roads

○ Never let a child on or near roads alone. Young children simply do not understand the dangers of traffic.

○ Hold your child's hand when you're out near roads. Walking reins can be useful for toddlers.

○ Always cross roads in the safest possible way. Use a pedestrian crossing if you can. Hold your child's hand firmly and talk about what you're doing every single time you cross.

Use the Green Cross Code. Begin to teach it early, and use it yourself. You can get information about the code from a road safety officer or RoSPA (address page 95).

Coping with accidents

You'll have to cope with some accidents while your child is young, mostly minor but maybe major.

○ Learn basic first aid, or revise what you already know. There is information on the following pages. You can also buy first aid books.

Better still, do a first aid course. Courses are run by both the British Red Cross (the Scottish Red Cross in Scotland) and the St John's Ambulance Association (the St Andrew's Ambulance Association in Scotland). These organisations have local branches. Look in your phone book, or contact the address on page 95.

○ Make sure you know what to do to get help in an emergency. See inside back cover.

Emergency first aid

In an emergency, don't panic. Try to keep calm. The child's life may depend on it, and calmness will help to comfort the child.

The really important things to check immediately are breathing, consciousness and bleeding.

1. Check breathing

If the child has stopped breathing, check the airway is clear, then give mouth-to-mouth resuscitation (the kiss of life) immediately. Every second counts.

Mouth-to-mouth resuscitation

1. First check the airway is clear. Use your finger to clear the child's mouth of any dirt, vomit etc. Then bend the head back with one hand and push the jaw upwards with the other hand. This lifts the tongue off the back of the throat.

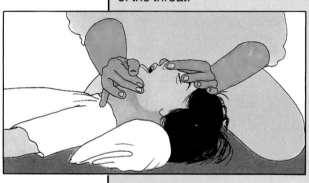

2. Squeeze the nostrils together, put your mouth completely over the child's mouth, and blow gently. See that the chest rises as you blow in.

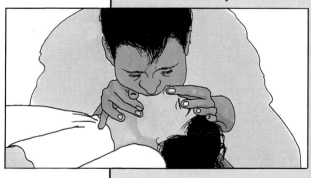

3. Take your mouth away and let the air come out of the child's chest.

4. Repeat this about 15 times a minute. Keep on until the child starts to breathe again.

5. Then gently place the child in the 'recovery' position (see opposite).

Note: With babies and children under 2 years old, it may be easier to breathe into the mouth and nose at the same time.

If, after several breaths given mouth-to-mouth, the child is still very pale or a blue/grey colour, then the heart may have stopped. If you think the heart has stopped, give heart massage as well as mouth-to-mouth resuscitation.

Heart massage

1. Lay the child on his/her back on the floor. Kneel by the child.

2. Press on the lower half of the child's breast bone. Use moderate pressure for a young child and even less for a baby. Press about once every second, quicker for a baby.

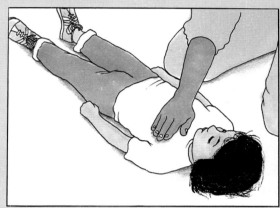

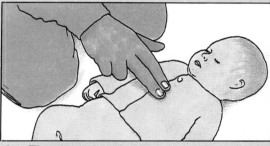

3. The child will not start breathing until after the heart has started beating. So after pressing 5 times, stop the heart massage and give a breath by mouth-to-mouth resuscitation. For babies and children under 2 years, it may be easier to breathe into the mouth and nose at the same time.

If there is another person with you, get them to do the breathing while you do the heart massage, stopping every 5 seconds to let the other person fill up the child's lungs.

4. Once the heart has started beating, keep on with mouth-to-mouth resuscitation until the breathing starts again.

5. Then gently place the child in the 'recovery' position (see opposite).

2. Check consciousness

It is dangerous for an unconscious child to lie on his/her back because the throat can be blocked by the tongue or by vomit. So if the child is unconscious or very drowsy, place him or her in the 'recovery' position.

Recovery position

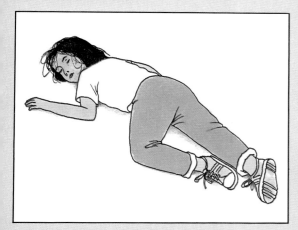

Turn the child half way over onto his or her front, with the underneath arm behind and the upper arm bent in front. Bend the upper leg so that it is at right angles to the trunk. Turn the face towards the ground with the neck back so that the tongue falls forward and the child can breathe.

If you think the child's back or neck may be broken, don't move the child unless you have to. Get expert help immediately.

Never leave an unconscious child alone unless you have to. The child may stop breathing or choke.

3. Check bleeding

If there's severe bleeding, press firmly on the wound using a pad of clean cloth (if available) or your fingers. Keep pressing until the bleeding stops.

4. Dial 999

If you need help, phone for an ambulance. Somebody else may be able to do this for you.

Broken bones

1. Don't move the child if you think the neck or spine may be injured. Get expert help.

2. For other broken bones, if the child has to be moved, be very gentle.

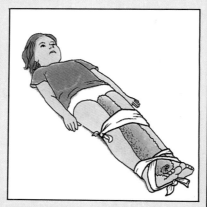

If it's a leg that's broken and the child has to be moved, tie the leg gently but firmly to the uninjured leg before moving the child. Put some padding between the legs.

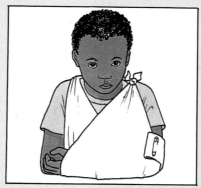

If it's an arm that's injured and if it can be moved, put it in a sling or support. Be gentle and comfort the child.

3. Call an ambulance, or take the child to hospital.

4. Don't give a child anything to drink after an accident if you think an anaesthetic may be needed later.

Burns and scalds

1. *Immediately* put the burn or scald under running cold water to reduce the heat in the skin. Do this for at least 10 minutes. If running water is not possible, immerse the burn or scald in cold water.

2. Cover the burn or scald with a clean, non-fluffy cloth like a clean cotton pillow case or linen tea towel. This cuts down the danger of infection.

3. If clothes are stuck to the skin, don't try to take them off.

4. Call an ambulance, or take the child to hospital. You should take a child to hospital for anything other than a very small burn or scald.

Don't put butter, oil or ointment on a burn or scald. It only has to be cleaned off again before treatment can be given.

Don't prick any blisters. You'll delay healing and let in germs.

Choking

1. Don't waste time trying to pick the object out with your fingers unless it's easy to get hold of. Probably it will be too far back and too slippery.

2. For babies and small children, quickly turn them upside down, holding them by the legs. Slap the back firmly between the shoulder blades. If the object doesn't come out, do it again.

If after several tries this hasn't worked, as a last resort give the baby's stomach a short sharp squeeze.

For bigger children, bend the child over the back of a settee or arm of a chair and give a good thump on the back, between the shoulder blades. If after several tries this hasn't worked, squeeze the stomach sharply by giving a quick, hard hug from behind.

Cuts

1. If there's a lot of bleeding, press firmly on the wound using a pad of clean cloth. If you have no cloth, use your fingers. Keep pressing until the bleeding stops. This may take 10 minutes or more.

2. Don't use a tourniquet or tie anything so tightly that it stops the circulation.

3. If possible, raise the injured limb. This helps to stop bleeding. But don't do this if you think the limb is broken.

4. Cover the wound with a clean dressing if you can find one. If you can't, don't cover the wound.

5. Then call an ambulance or take the child to hospital.

6. Ask your doctor about a tetanus injection.

Don't give a child anything to drink after an accident if you think an anaesthetic may be needed later.

Poisoning

Pills and medicines

1. If you're not sure whether the child has swallowed something, spend a minute or two looking for the missing pills. Check they haven't rolled under a chair, for example.

2. If you still think something has been swallowed, take the child straight away to your doctor or to hospital – whichever is quickest.

3. If possible, take with you the container (or its label) and a sample of whatever you think has been swallowed.

Don't give salt and water to make the child sick. Large amounts of salt can be dangerous.

Household and garden chemicals

1. If you think something poisonous has been swallowed, calm the child as much as you can. You will do this better if you can keep calm yourself. But act quickly: get the child to hospital.

If possible, take with you the container (or its label) and a sample of whatever you think has been swallowed.

2. If the child is in pain, or if there is any staining, soreness or blistering around the mouth, then the child has probably swallowed something corrosive. Take a few moments to give the child a glass of milk or water to sip. This dilutes the poison and helps to lessen the burning. Get the child to hospital quickly.

Shock

1. If pale, unwell or feeling faint after an accident, help the child to lie down.

2. If a lot of blood has been lost, keep the head down and raise the legs. This makes more blood go to the head. But don't do this if you suspect a head injury or broken leg.

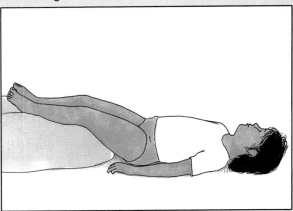

3. Keep the child covered up and warm but not too hot.

Don't give a child anything to drink after an accident if you think an anaesthetic may be needed later.

Suffocation

1. Quickly take away whatever is causing the suffocation.

2. If the child has stopped breathing, give mouth-to-mouth resuscitation (see page 66).

A child should go to hospital after an accident if he or she:

○ is or has been unconscious

○ is vomiting or drowsy

○ is bleeding from the ears

○ has stopped breathing at some stage

○ may have internal injuries

○ complains of severe pain anywhere.

If you are worried or uncertain about a child's injuries, get a doctor's advice. Go to the accident and emergency department of the nearest hospital with a children's unit, or to a local doctor, whichever is quickest. Not all hospitals have an accident and emergency department, so check in advance where your nearest one is. Your health visitor will be able to tell you.

See inside back cover for how to get help in an emergency.

5. Your own life

"I can't say I always put them first. My mum says the kids always come first, but I don't see it like that. It's not just the children, it's us too, it's the *family*. And Sean and I are just as much a part of the family as the kids are."

"Sometimes I feel like a steamroller's been over me. And I think when you get like that, you can't be the sort of parent you want to be. It's give, give, give all the time, and sometimes you've got to give something to yourself."

"People say, 'How's the baby doing?' And I want to say, 'Well, she's okay, but do you want to know how *I'm* feeling?' "

"I think Dave thinks I've got an easy life, you know, just being at home all day. He thinks I can just suit myself and do what I want to do. I get very angry, because there are days when I'd give anything to be walking out of the house like he does."

(A father) "I suppose I'd thought that having a kid wouldn't change that much for me. Obviously it was going to make a difference financially, with Linda giving up work. Apart from that, I'd thought it was Linda's life that was going to change and that I'd be going on much the same as before. Who was I kidding?"

Being a parent is hard work. It's hard on you physically, and hard emotionally too.

All parents go through times of feeling extremely tired, not just because of lack of sleep but also because of having to cope with a different, often stressful sort of life. Any sort of change can be tiring, and a baby brings enormous changes. In fact, children *go on* bringing changes; and you have to go on adapting.

A lot of parents also feel that, in the midst of loving and caring for their children, they lose sight of themselves and their own lives. Sometimes it seems impossible to fit into your life anything that's for you. Sometimes just *caring* for yourself at the same time as caring for the family seems out of the question.

But unless you do care for yourself, you won't cope so well. Keeping healthy, feeling all right about yourself and your life, being you as a person as well as you as a parent, are all very important. If you care for yourself, you're more likely to enjoy being a parent, and more likely to keep on top of a very hard job.

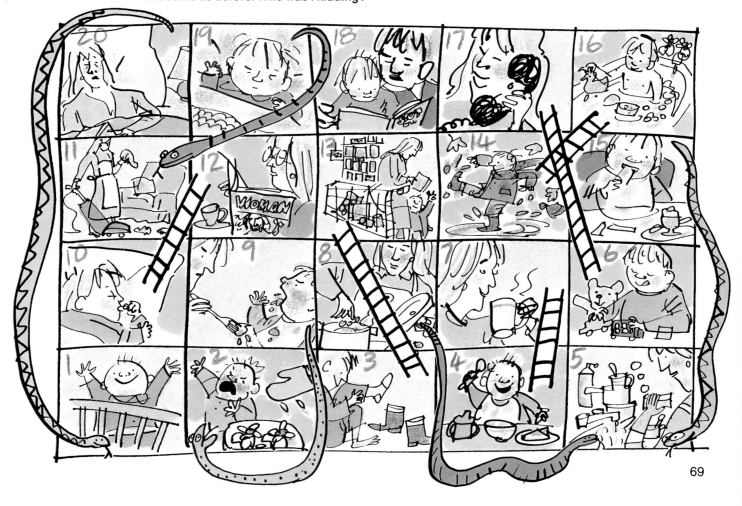

Keeping healthy

"You get so used to managing without sleep and, you know, grabbing something to eat, it doesn't matter what, and just rushing on from one thing to the next. It's crazy, really. I'll spend ages feeding the baby, but I don't feed myself properly at all. I'm anxious for her to sleep, but once she's off, I don't think about getting some sleep myself. Then I wonder why I'm feeling so rough . . ."

"You have to be quite tough with yourself. Because you tend to put things off. You say, 'Oh well, I'll cook a proper meal tomorrow', or 'I'll start doing exercises again when I'm not so tired', or whatever. You get to think it doesn't really matter and you just neglect yourself. I need my doctor to write me a prescription saying 'look after yourself'."

Looking after small children often gets in the way of looking after yourself. But you'll survive parenthood much better if you can keep yourself fit and healthy. If you can only get something like the sleep you need, eat properly and get some sort of exercise, you will not only manage better but also feel better. Morale always drops when you're tired and run down.

Try to see that your own health (and happiness) really matters. Here is a basic survival guide.

Eating

Eat well. Look back to the guidelines for 'Feeding the family' on pages 46-49. If you can follow these, you'll be eating a healthy diet. And if you eat a healthy diet, you'll be fitter and have more energy.

When there isn't time, or you feel too tired to cook much, try to find quick and easy food that is still nutritious. See page 49 for some ideas.

If you feel you need to lose weight, cut down further on fat and sugar. Just as simple, eat less. If you're choosing the right sorts of foods, then eating smaller meals, maybe more often, is a better way of getting your weight down and keeping it down than any crash diet. So, for example, when you eat with the children, use a small plate like theirs – and don't eat up their leftovers. If you don't need the food, it's just as much wasted in you as in the bin.

Be careful when you shop. If you don't *buy* the foods that will make you fat, you won't be able to eat them – and the whole family will be better for fewer fatty and sugary foods.

Don't start to diet while breast feeding. You need calories to produce milk. If you follow the guidelines on pages 46-49, you won't put on weight. In fact, you are quite likely to lose some.

Exercise

Try to get some exercise. Often exercise seems to demand time and energy you haven't got. Often, when you're feeling tired, it seems like the last thing you need. But exercise relaxes you, helps your body recover after childbirth, keeps you fit *and* makes you feel better in yourself.

In the early months after your baby's birth, keep up the postnatal exercises you should have been taught. Stick at them. They will strengthen vital muscles and improve your shape. Two important exercises are described on page 73.

If you need to strengthen your will power, you could join a postnatal exercise class. Find out if your local maternity unit has a class run by an obstetric physiotherapist, or ask your health visitor about other local classes.

Later on, exercise is still important but becomes more difficult to get. It may help if you stop thinking of exercise as something you have to make special time for and start thinking about it as how you stand and sit and

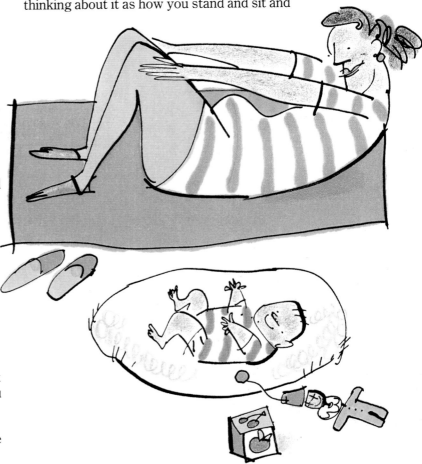

move about every single day. You're probably already very energetic. You can build on that by teaching yourself to be energetic in the right sort of way, not straining your body but making the muscles and joints work like they're supposed to work. So, for example:

○ Push the pram or buggy briskly, back straight. Get out for walks as much as you can.

○ Play energetic games with older children, making yourself run about as well as them. Find outdoor space if there's no space at home.

○ Run upstairs. You probably find yourself going up and down a hundred times a day in any case. Try to look on it as good exercise!

○ Squat down to pick things up from the floor. This is also something you're likely to be doing a lot. If you squat rather than stoop, bending your knees and keeping your back straight, you will improve your thigh muscles. You will also avoid damaging your back.

This sort of exercise can go on all the time. But you might also think about going to an exercise class, or doing some exercises at home, perhaps with a friend. Get children to join in. Children are usually welcome at classes run for mothers. Ask your health visitor about local classes.

Note: if you have or have had a bad back or any similar problem, you do need to be careful about what exercise you do. Tell whoever runs your class about the problem.

Sleep

You need sleep, but few parents get the sleep they need. Make sure you get what you can. Sometimes this means putting sleep before other things. An hour's sleep in the day, if it's possible, could keep you going.

If you go through times when you simply cannot get enough sleep, at least look for ways of resting. Reading your child a story, for example, or watching a TV programme together.

It's important to deal with tiredness, and not let it get you down. See page 74 for ways of coping.

Time for yourself

Time for yourself and time to relax is just as important for your health as eating a good diet. Looking after children is often stressful, however much you enjoy it. Stress that goes on 24 hours a day isn't good for anyone. See page 75 for some ideas.

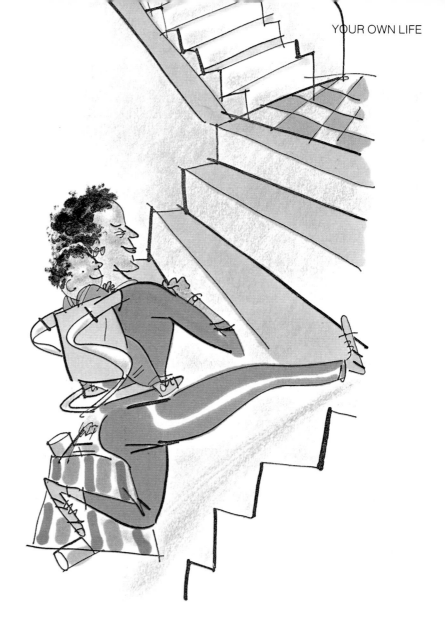

Your body after childbirth

"I just don't like myself any more. My whole body's completely changed."

"I think everyone assumes that after the first month or so, you're back to normal again. But I know from talking to friends that I'm not the only one to feel like I'm anything but normal."

"A frump. That's what I am. But where's the time to do anything about it?"

Having a baby does change your body and a lot of women don't like the change. Some are luckier than others, but if you feel that your body is not the way you would like it to be, you are certainly not alone.

Yet to like yourself, you need to feel all right about your body.

That may mean accepting that your body is never going to be quite the same as it was

71

before. There are some things, like stretch marks, which are always going to be there – though they will fade. If you can only stop wishing you were the same as before, or that you could change what can't be changed, you'll start to get on with yourself better.

On the other hand, you don't have to accept what you don't like about your body if there *is* something you can do about it. And if doing something is going to make you feel better, it's worth making time to do it. For example, if you've got stretch marks *and* a baggy, bulging stomach, then exercises to improve your stomach muscles (see 'curl ups' opposite) will flatten the bulge, and the stretch marks won't seem so bad. If you have the feeling, especially when you're tired, that you're 'dropping out' underneath, then pelvic floor exercises (see opposite) will help.

Quite small things can boost morale. For example, if it makes you feel more yourself to paint your toe nails, then make time to do it. Maybe for you that's even more important than 20 minutes extra sleep. The same goes for any of the small ways in which you can give your body attention. You won't have time for much. But putting one thing at the top of the list and doing just that, might make all the difference. It depends on the kind of person you are. If you don't mind the way you are, don't let other people tell you that you should.

Physical problems

"You think you're the only person in the world with this problem, and you feel embarrassed and, you know, almost a bit ashamed, as though somehow it's your fault. So you just go on and try to forget about it or hope it will go. And when it doesn't, you get really fed up. It was only because I got talking to a friend, and we found out we both felt the same, it was only then that I started to think, well, maybe I can do something about this. And because there were two of us, we had a bit more courage and could back each other up."

"You have your postnatal check, and then that's it. After that, it seems like everything is laid on to keep the children healthy, and you take *them* to the clinic or the doctor or whatever, but there's nothing for you. I think just like there are clinics and regular checks for children, there ought to be clinics for mothers too. Because as it is, you sit there thinking, well, should I go to the doctor, or where? And you don't go because there's not enough time anyway."

A lot of women do have physical problems – either as a result of labour and birth, or because of the kind of work involved in caring for young children, or both. Problems like some sort of infection which keeps coming back, a bad back, a leaky bladder, painful intercourse, are much more common than people think. These sorts of problems can get you down, and some get worse if they're not seen to.

Helping yourself

It may be that you can do something for yourself. For example, a weak perineum (the muscles around your bladder, vagina and back passage) is often the cause of a leaky bladder and can be improved by pelvic floor exercises. A bad back can also be helped by exercise, and by learning to move in a way that avoids strain.

Pelvic floor exercise

The muscles of the pelvic floor form a hammock underneath the pelvis to support the bladder, womb and bowel. You use these muscles when you pass water, empty your bowels, and when you make love. Often they are stretched during pregnancy, labour and birth. If you can get them back into shape (and keep them that way), you're less likely to have a leaky bladder, and more likely to enjoy intercourse.

You can do this exercise sitting or standing, when you're washing up, queueing in the supermarket, watching television – anywhere. You ought to do it for the rest of your life. It's an exercise that's just as important for older women as younger.

○ Squeeze shut your back passage, close up and draw in your vagina, close your front passage, all at the same time. Hold while you count to four, then let go.

It helps to imagine you're stopping a bowel movement, holding in a tampon, stopping yourself passing water. In fact, you can practise while on the toilet, trying to stop and start the flow of urine. You may be able to stop and start, or you may just slow down the stream. Keep trying.

Curl ups

This exercise helps to prevent or ease back pain. It also firms up your stomach and closes the gap in the abdominal muscles that opens up during pregnancy.

○ Lie on the floor (rather than your bed) with knees bent up high so your feet are flat on the floor.

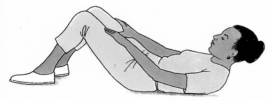

○ Pull your stomach in and gradually lift your head and shoulders, reaching for your knees with your hands. Then lower back down very slowly.

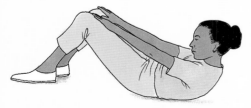

Begin this exercise gently and build up.

To ease back problems

○ Always sit with your back well supported and straight. Use a pillow or cushion behind your waist.

○ Kneel or squat to do low-level jobs – like bathing your baby or picking things up off the floor. Avoid bending your back. Make your knees work instead. Change nappies on a waist-level surface or, once your baby starts to roll, try sitting on the floor, legs wide apart and your baby lying between them.

○ To lift weights, like a carrycot or an older child, bend your knees, keep your back straight, and hold the weight close to your body. Make your thigh muscles work as you lift.

○ Try to keep a straight back when you push a pram or buggy or carry your baby in a sling.

Getting help

It may be that you need medical advice. Try to get to your doctor rather than ignoring a problem. If you can, arrange to go without your child or children with you so you can talk more easily. Or take someone with you who can wait with your child in the waiting room. Besides asking about treatment, you may also want to ask whether there is anything you can do for yourself, either to cure the problem, or ease it, or prevent it cropping up again.

If a visit to your doctor doesn't give you the solution you're looking for, you may want to ask to be referred to a specialist. You can also look for other help. Use as many sources of information as you can find, including books and magazines. Talk to other women. Solutions that have worked for them may not be right for you. But just talking may help you decide what is the best thing for you to try. And it's always comforting to discover you're not the only one with a particular problem.

In some areas there are women's groups, run by women for women, often with a special interest in women's health. You can get a lot of information and moral support from these groups. Ask your health visitor if there is a local group, or look on noticeboards in places like community centres, libraries, clinics, health centres.

How you feel

Tiredness

"I think the tiredness is the worst thing. It goes on and on. And you've got no choice, you've got to keep going. So you feel sort of trapped. And after a bit, it gets you down, feeling so tired all the time."

(A father) **"You come in from work and you start right in on another job. And then when you've got them off to bed, there are still other things you've got to do. So you drop into bed and there's been no breathing space. You're probably up in the night as well. And then you get up the next morning and start it all over again."**

Most of the time parents just live with tiredness. But when the tiredness begins to make you feel low, bad-tempered, unable to cope and certainly unable to enjoy things, you've got to find ways of getting more sleep – or at least more rest. Just one day, one night, one week, could help.

○ Get to bed early, really early, say for a week. If you can't sleep when you get to bed, do something relaxing for half an hour beforehand, whether that's exercise, or soaking in a bath, or watching television.

○ Most parents find themselves dropping off when they put their children to bed. You could let yourself do just that and sleep for an hour or so.

○ Sleep when your baby sleeps. Rest when (if) your child has a daytime rest, or is at playgroup or nursery school. Arrange for a relative or friend to take your child for a while, *not* so that you can get the jobs done but so you can sleep. Take turns with other parents to give yourself time to rest. Set an alarm if you're worried about sleeping too long.

○ If you can, share getting up in the night with your partner. Take alternate nights or weeks. If you're on your own, you might think of arranging for your child to sleep at a friend's or relative's house every now and then.

○ Look at pages 19 and 43 for other ways of coping with disturbed nights.

○ Read on. Tiredness often comes from stress. If you can do something about the stress, you may be able to cope better, even without more sleep.

Stress

"They make me so angry. You wouldn't believe how wound up I get. Most of the time I sort of swallow it, but there are other times when they must hear me shouting down the other end of the block. I sometimes wonder whether other mothers get like that, because you see them walking down the street and they certainly don't look the way I feel."

"It's the two of them. What one wants the other doesn't want. When I'm getting the little one off to sleep, the older one suddenly decides he needs the potty. You can't seem to do right by both of them. You're split in two, and there's no let-up, it's the whole time."

"I wouldn't really call it stress. But it's hard to explain to someone who isn't a parent how, even when you're enjoying it, there's this sort of constant drain on you. You think about them all the time, you have to. You have to think *for* them all the time. Even when I'm out at work, I have to think about getting back on time, and remembering to tell the childminder something, and buying something for tea . . . "

"It gets so frustrating. I wake up in the morning and think, 'Right, what have I got today?' And then I give myself a great big long list of all the things I've got to do, and if I can't get them done in that day, I get really narked about it."

Small children can put you under a lot of strain just by the way they are. They ask a lot of you, and there's a limit to what you can ask of them. But perhaps the greatest stress comes from coping with the rest of life *at the same time* as coping with a baby or small child. You can spend a whole day trying your utmost to get one job done but never managing to fit it in. Just as you start on it, your baby wakes up, or a nappy needs changing, or your child wants attention. Sometimes you can feel as though life is completely out of control. And if you're not the sort of person who can take things as they come and not mind about what is or isn't done, you can get to feel very tense and frustrated.

Stress also comes from worry and unhappiness – maybe to do with the place you live, money, relationships, or just a lot of small but important things.

You may not be able to change the way your children are or the life you lead. But you may be able to do something about the stress. It's a matter of finding solutions that are right for you.

○ Make time for yourself, to do exactly what *you* want to do. Your partner or a grandparent might be able to give you time. Or 'swap' children with a friend so that each week one of you has an hour or two off.

○ See other people: it does take the pressure off. Try a mother and baby, or parent and toddler group. Ask your health visitor or other parents about local groups. Or, if you're not keen on organised groups, get together with people you meet at the clinic, playgroup or nursery school.

○ Make time to be with your partner, even if only to fall asleep together in front of the television. Relationships can go wrong when you're tense and tired and never seem to see each other.

○ Talking about the stress you're feeling can help to get rid of it, at least for a while. Talking with your partner isn't always best. Sometimes it's good to talk with people outside the family. But if you and your partner can understand how each other is feeling, it may help you support each other better.

○ Take some sort of physical exercise. Physical activity relieves tension, and though you may feel you are active to the point of exhaustion, you're probably not active in a way that relaxes you. Swimming is good, relaxing exercise. If you take your child with you, try to have someone else with you too, so that you get a chance to swim. Or think of joining some kind of exercise class. This means you meet people too. Ask your health visitor about classes in your area.

○ For you, relaxation may come from just doing something that you enjoy, can do for

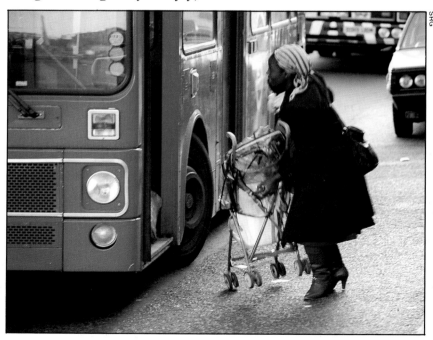

half an hour in the evening, and will put other things out of your mind for a while. A bath, maybe, or time to look at a magazine or the television. Do whatever will wind you down. You may have to *make* yourself do it.

○ Make the very most of all the help you can find. And give up a bit. You can't do everything. Try to believe it really doesn't matter.

Look back to Chapter 3 'How do you cope?' for more suggestions.

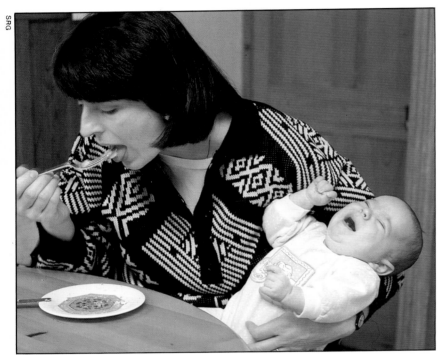

Feeling low

"I wouldn't say I was depressed. But I do feel fed up, and just, well, unhappy, I suppose. I mean, it's so disappointing. Other people think you must be enjoying it all, but the fact is, I'm not. This old lady walked by me in the street the other day when I was out with the buggy, and she was smiling at the baby and she said, 'It's the best time in your life, dear. You make the most of it.' Well, I'm not feeling it's the best time in my life, but I know what she means, and I feel guilty that I'm not enjoying it."

You're not unusual if you go through patches of feeling low. No job is all pleasure and satisfaction and being a parent is no exception. In fact, just as the good times are especially good, the bad times can also be especially bad.

But knowing it's normal to feel low doesn't make the feeling any better. What might help is to read through the suggestions given elsewhere in this chapter. Health problems, tiredness, lack of time for yourself, feeling under stress or just feeling lonely, can all get

you down. Doing something to deal with one or two of your own needs can lift you up a lot.

Try, too, to talk to somebody about the way you feel. You may want to talk to people close to you, or, if you find them friendly and sympathetic, your health visitor or doctor. Talking to your partner can be important, for both your sakes. When you're feeling unhappy, it's easy to blame it on the person you're living with, and expect them to do something about it. But they can't begin to know how to help unless you give them a few clues. In any case, it isn't easy to live with somebody who's feeling miserable, and it helps to understand.

Whoever you talk to, try to sort out the reasons for your feelings. You might then be able to sort out what you can do to help yourself feel better. And, because it is often quite hard to help yourself, try to find someone who'll give you some support. If you tell somebody else you're going to do something, or ask them to do it with you, you're more likely to carry it through.

Feeling depressed

"I think you get to the point when you can't see the good side of anything. And when you get like that, nothing has much point. It didn't seem worth getting up in the mornings, and once I had got up, there didn't seem any point in bothering to get dressed. And it went on like that the whole day. Everything was too much effort. I'd got no energy, no desire to do anything."

"It's like you're kicking against everything that's happening to you. You feel out of control, underneath it all. The baby was too much, the flat was all wrong, my husband never did or said anything right . . . I was angry inside myself, all the time."

"I don't think anybody knew how I was feeling because I never said anything and when I was out of the house I wasn't that bad. You sort of carry on somehow, and people don't know what you're like when you're on your own. You hardly realise yourself what's happening to you or how bad things are."

A lot of people talk about being depressed but mean that they're miserable or unhappy in some way. True depression is something different. It's feeling hopeless, about yourself and all that's happening to you. The hopelessness can make you angry. But often you feel too tired even for anger. It can seem as though there's no answer and no end to the way you're feeling.

Sometimes this kind of depression has a physical cause – hormone imbalance, for example, or exhaustion. But for lots of parents, and for mothers especially, depression comes from a combination of a lot of things which together make life difficult – living in the wrong sort of place, having no money, feeling under stress, feeling no good as a parent.

This kind of depression is like an illness. Nothing seems worth doing, so doing anything as demanding as caring for a baby or child becomes a real struggle. Both for yourself and for the family, it's important to get help.

See your doctor, or health visitor, or both. However difficult it is, try to explain how you feel. Take someone with you if this would help. Make it clear that you're not talking about just feeling low but something more worrying than that.

Just talking, and getting your doctor's or health visitor's support, may be enough to see you through. But having worked out with you what might be causing the depression, your doctor may be able to suggest other help, maybe referring you elsewhere.

If hormonal causes are likely, and you are taking the contraceptive pill, then a change of pill, or a change to another kind of contraceptive, may well help. If the depression is bad, you may be offered hormone treatment, or anti-depressant drugs. Think carefully about whether this is what you want. Discuss it fully with your doctor. It's your decision, but to make that decision, you need information. Anti-depressant drugs can sometimes help for a time while other solutions are worked out. But they need to be used with care and may take time to work. Tranquillisers are often offered but don't help depression and can be habit-forming if taken for longer than two or three months.

No drug can substitute for talking the problem through and finding the right sort of continuing support. Two organisations which offer help are the Association for Post-Natal Illness, and MAMA, the Meet-a-Mum Association (addresses on page 94). Both give help through other mothers who have been depressed themselves and know what it's like.

Remember that what is called postnatal depression can happen a long time after the birth of a baby.

Alcohol may appear to help you relax and unwind. In fact it's a depressant, affecting judgment, self-control and co-ordination. If you're tired and run down, it affects these even more. So watch how much and when you drink. Never mix alcohol with anti-depressants or tranquillisers.

Loneliness

"At first you hardly notice it. You're bound up with the baby, and there's so much that's new, and such a lot to do. So you don't bother to meet up with people. Then you wake up one morning and you've got a whole day ahead of you and you know you're not going to see or talk to anybody, the whole day through."

"At home in Pakistan, there's a lot of visiting, lots of people about, and children can go anywhere. Here there isn't so much coming and going. You can feel very isolated."

"When I was working, there were lots of people to talk to and I had all the company I needed. Now I haven't got any of that, I really miss it. And I think I've lost confidence. I don't find it so easy to talk to people."

Lots of mothers feel lonely. Especially after the birth of a first baby, many find that they're cut off from old friends but it's difficult to make new ones. Getting out to see people, even if you've got people to see, is often an effort. Meeting new people takes confidence.

But loneliness can make you miserable. Often it has a lot to do with depression. Certainly any problem is twice as big when you're on your own with it.

Take courage: try to make some contacts.

○ Chat with other mothers at your baby or child health clinic. If you find it hard to start a conversation, ask your health visitor for information about mother and baby groups, parent and toddler groups, playgroups etc. These may be advertised on the clinic noticeboard.

○ Your health visitor should also be able to tell you about local groups, or might be able to put you in touch with other mothers living near you.

○ MAMA, Home-Start, the National Childbirth Trust and many of the other organisations listed on page 94, run local groups where you can meet other people, chat, relax and get a lot of support.

○ You may want to find a group of people with the same background and culture as yours. See 'Local groups' on page 87 for information.

○ Some mothers find the answer to feeling lonely and cut off is to take a job. It's not always easy to find the right sort of work with the right sort of hours, or to make child care arrangements. But if you feel that work outside the home could help you, turn to page 80 for more information.

Relationships

"We argue a lot. There seems so much more to argue about. And because very often we're overtired anyway, and frustrated in lots of ways because we haven't got the freedom we had, sometimes the arguments are really bad. When you're tired, you say things you don't mean, you hit out that much more easily."

"There's a lot of pressure, it's true. I think we've had to learn a lot, and learn it fast, about how to get on when there's so much to cope with. But then, there's a lot we both enjoy, and more to share, really."

Relationships are often strained by parenthood, no matter what they were like before. Quite a lot of couples go through some shaky times while children are young. Knowing this is normal, try to recognise the strains that are pulling you apart, talk about them if you can, and do what you can to see each other through.

It may be that you can do some quite practical things. When you're both tired and overworked, with little or no time for yourselves, you're almost bound to have rows. If you can only get more sleep, take a bit of time together, or maybe give each other time alone, it could make a big difference.

It's sharing the work and responsibility which is perhaps the most difficult thing. Very often one partner feels they're carrying an unfair burden, and even in the best relationships there can be a lot of bitterness. A lot of couples find they disagree about how to bring up children. Behaviour that one parent sees as wrong, the other sees as all right, or even funny. There is really no answer to this sort of problem except to talk about it. If you can talk about the way you feel without arguing or accusing each other, you may be able to sort out a better way of working together.

If you feel your relationship is really breaking down, get help. RELATE (National Marriage Guidance) has local branches where you can talk to someone in confidence, either with your partner or alone. Counselling is offered on all sorts of relationship difficulties: you don't have to be married to contact marriage guidance. To find your local branch, look under RELATE or 'Marriage Guidance' in your phone book, or write to the address on page 94.

The problems for single parents are different. It can be hard, if not impossible, to have any kind of social life, relationships or sex life while your child is small, and loneliness is often a problem. Loneliness can still be a problem even if you feel that the last thing you want is a relationship with one other person. Look back to page 77 for some ways round this.

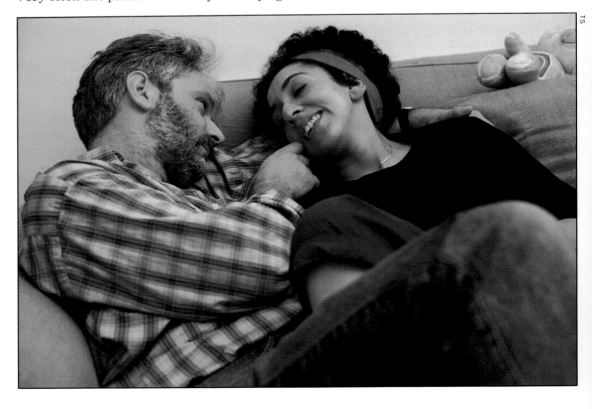

Sex

"I couldn't think about it. My mind was on the baby. And it sounds bad, but all my feelings seemed to be taken up by the baby too. And that caused a lot of difficulty for a while. I did feel bad about it, as though it was my fault. But you can't make love as an obligation, can you? I mean, you can, but it's not really any good for either of you."

"A chance would be a fine thing. Anyway, when you do get the chance, you're too tired."

(A father) "It's not talked about, is it? Except as a sort of joke. So you don't know if you've got a problem or not. At first, Paula found it hurt, and it put us both off and frightened us a bit. We were worried because we didn't know whether that was normal."

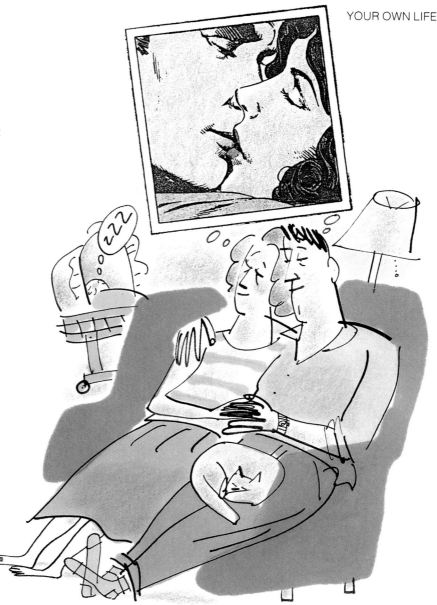

Babies and small children don't make for an easy sex life. Often you're tired, maybe too strained, and opportunities are limited. This hardly matters if both you and your partner are content. But if sex is a problem in any way at all, it's important to look at what you can do. Unhappy sex, or just lack of it, can cause a lot of frustration and worry, and can really strain relationships.

How soon you start making love again after the birth is up to you. It may not be a problem. But a lot of women do have feelings that put them off. You may feel worried about the state of your body (especially your vagina). You may be worried about getting pregnant again. You may feel unattractive, or sore.

Men can face problems too. Tiredness apart, a father's sexual feelings will probably be much the same as before his baby's birth. But many men worry about what is right for their partner, are unsure what to do, and feel worried and frustrated.

○ Make time to relax together. There's little point trying to make love when your minds are on anything but each other.

○ Sort out contraception. It is possible to become pregnant again soon after the birth of a baby, even if you are breast feeding, and even if you haven't re-started your periods. So if you don't want to conceive again quickly, you need to use some kind of contraception from the start.

Contraception is usually discussed before leaving hospital after the birth, and at the postnatal check-up. But you can go at any time, before or after your check-up, to your own doctor or family planning clinic, or talk with your health visitor.

○ If penetration hurts, find other ways of loving for a while and take your time. Massage is relaxing and brings you close. If penetration is still painful two months or so after the birth, go to your doctor for a check.

○ Use extra lubrication, such as lubricating jelly. Hormone changes after birth may mean your vagina is drier for a while.

○ Many women are worried about what may have happened to their bodies during birth. It may help you to have a good look at your perineum (the area around your vagina). Use a mirror in a good light. It may also help to feel your vagina with your fingers.

○ If your baby sleeps in the same room as you, you may have to move either yourselves or your baby before you can relax enough to make love.

○ Don't rush. Take time. But if patience runs out or problems can't be solved, go to your doctor, health visitor or family planning clinic for help.

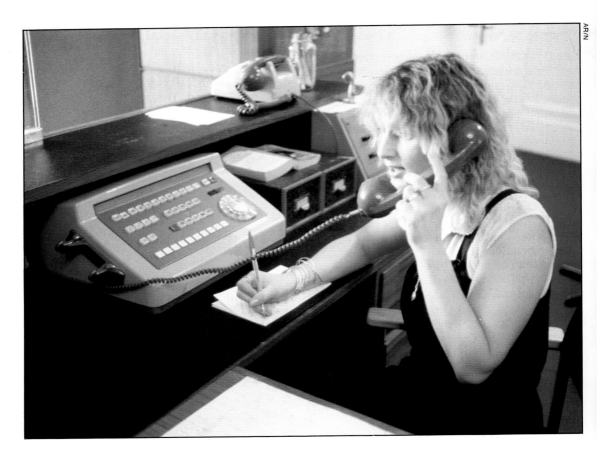

Going back to work

"At first, I hated leaving her. It was much more upsetting than I'd thought – but more for me than for her, really. I'm better about it now, especially as time goes by and I can see that she's happy and well looked after and I've got to know and like the person who cares for her. But I don't think you can ever feel completely right about it. So you just have to live with that and get on with it."

"There's no doubt it's hard work. I mean, there's no evenings off, because it's then that we have to get all the jobs done round the house. To my mind, families where there's one parent at home all the time have it very easy in comparison."

"I enjoy the job. It's nothing much, but it earns money we need, and it gets me out and makes me do things I'd not do otherwise. I think I'm a better parent for doing it. I like having contact with people other than mothers. And Darren gets to meet other children, and he thrives on that."

You may not have a choice about whether or not you work. But if you do have a choice, think hard. Paid work, on top of work at home, can bring benefits, even if the pay is not much. It can also make life tough.

You need to think –

– about the arrangements you'll have to make and whether these will work for everyone involved. Arrangements have to be as simple as possible to work smoothly. If they don't work smoothly, there's a lot of strain. You also have to be reasonably sure they'll go on working over time.

– about the money. You may want to work for other reasons, but if you're working for the money, you'll have to weigh up earnings against childcare costs, or perhaps against living on benefits.

– about when to start. The ideal is probably *either* when your child is still very young (say, under eight months) *or* when your child is three or more. A two year old who has never been left before can find separation very difficult and may take a long time to adjust.

– about what life will be like for everybody in the family day to day. It's worth thinking in advance about, for example, how and when you're going to do the shopping, how you're going to cope when your child is ill, and so on. If you can count on some help and support, it makes it much easier.

It may help to talk to other working mothers. But also try to decide what's right for you and your family.

Child care

The amount of day care that's provided for children varies a lot from one area to another. In some areas, there is very little. Your health visitor may be able to give you information. Many areas also produce handbooks listing local facilities for under-fives, including child care. Ask at your social services department, local library or citizens advice bureau.

Unless you can afford to employ somebody to look after your child/children in your own home, or are lucky enough to have, say, your mother living nearby and able to take over, your options may be a childminder, a nursery, or sharing/group care.

A childminder, usually a mother herself, looks after a small number of other people's children in her own home. Anybody paid to look after children under five in this way for more than two hours a day should apply to register as a childminder with the local social services department. This doesn't apply to close relatives, but it does apply to friends or neighbours. A childminder is usually registered to care for not more than three children under five, including any of her own. Registered childminders are visited by the social services to check that their homes are suitable and that they can give a good standard of care. So if you go to a childminder you don't know, it's worth asking if she is registered. You can ask to see her certificate.

You should be able to get names of childminders with vacancies from your social services department. Other working mothers will also be able to tell you about childminders. If you don't already know mothers who use childminders, ask your health visitor to put you in touch.

Day nurseries run by local authorities are few and far between. They often have long waiting lists, and only a limited number of places for very young children. Priority is usually given to parents who, for one reason or another, are under a lot of stress and are unable to cope, to parents of handicapped children, and, sometimes, to working single parents. To get a place at a council nursery, apply to your social services department. Your need will then be assessed by a social worker.

There may be nurseries in your area run privately or on a community basis by parents themselves. These nurseries should be

> To contact your social services department, look in your phone book under the name of your local authority.
>
> In Scotland the social services department is called the social work department; in Northern Ireland it is the health and social services board.

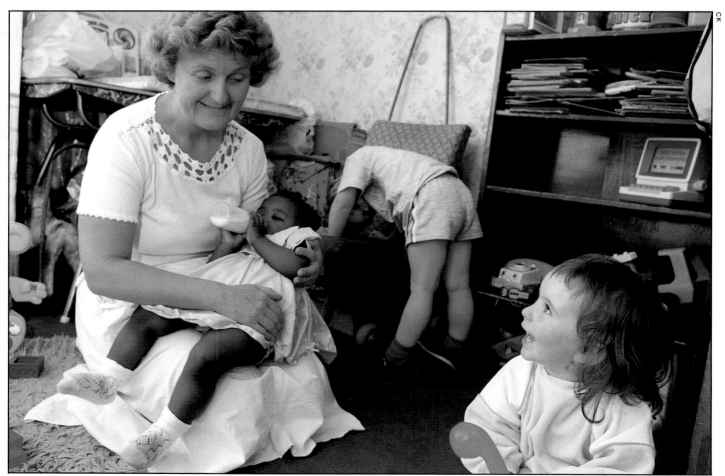

registered with the local authority and you can find out about them through your local social services department.

You may be lucky enough to have a nursery or crèche at your place of work. If one doesn't exist but there are a number of parents wanting and needing one, it's worth discussing the possibility with your employer. An organisation called Workplace Nurseries (address on page 94) can give information.

Sharing/group care means getting together with other parents with needs like your own and organising your own child care. This can work well if at least some of you work part-time. Your health visitor may be able to put you in touch with other parents who work or want to work and need child care. The National Childcare Campaign (address on page 94) supplies information about setting up group care.

The cost of child care

Costs vary. You will have to ask. The cost of a nursery place may depend on your income. It is up to you to agree pay with a childminder, but your social services department may guide you. The National Childminding Association (address on page 94) also gives advice. In some areas, childminding fees are subsidised for low-income or single-parent families.

Making it work

○ Before you decide on child care, visit the childminder/nursery, talk, and ask all the questions on your mind. Talk about hours, fees, what the fees cover, what happens during holidays, when there's illness or an emergency. Go through every detail of an arrangement to make sure there's every chance that it will work.

○ It helps if children can settle in gradually. If you can, start by leaving your child for short times and build up. This might mean starting to leave your child before you actually start your job.

○ Tell your childminder or nursery all about your child, his or her routine, likes and dislikes, and so on. When you leave or collect your child, try to make time to talk and find out how things are going.

○ There may be special worries you want to talk about. For example, if your child is going to be one of very few black children at a mainly white nursery, you may want to talk to the people in charge about how they will handle this and perhaps make some suggestions yourself. A white childminder may well not know, for example, how to do a black child's hair. And if this is important to you, it's right to talk about it.

○ Support and reassure your child in every way you can. The early weeks are likely to be difficult for both of you. A regular routine, and a handover that's as smooth as possible, both help. Expect crying when you leave, maybe for longer than just the early weeks, but remember the crying usually stops once you've gone. (You can ask how long it has gone on.) It's best not to linger long, nor to leave and then go back. Try to keep promises about when you'll return and explain to older children when that will be.

○ Chat with older children about the daily routine, about the person or people caring for them, about what they've done while away from you. Try to show it's a part of normal life and something to look forward to.

○ For you, do your best to keep on top. It helps to get into a routine, and you need to make time with your child part of that routine. A lot of other things will have to go, especially the housework – but *not* sleep or meals. Share out the work at home with your partner if you can, or get friends and neighbours to help.

○ Remember that, provided your child is well cared for, he or she is quite likely to benefit, and very *un*likely to suffer. Most children like having other children's company and thrive on it.

And don't lose sight of the benefits for you.

6. Help and support

There's no parent who doesn't need, at one time or another, some kind of help or support.

There's a wide range of help available, both through the services and through voluntary organisations and local groups. But it is often difficult to know where to find what you're looking for.

This section should help you track down the help you need.

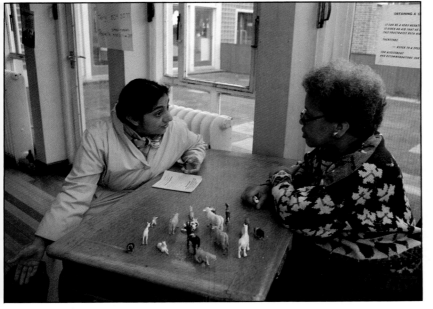

The services

Health services

Your community midwife looks after you in the early weeks at home with your baby. She can help with any problem to do with yourself or your baby and will give you a phone number to call at any time, day or night, if you need to.

Your health visitor usually makes her first visit sometime after your baby is ten days old. She can help at any time from then onwards. She is a qualified nurse who has had extra training to become a health visitor. Her role is to help families (especially families with babies and young children) avoid illness and keep healthy. She can help with problems or worries either to do with yourself or your child. She may visit you at home, or you can see her at your child health clinic, doctor's surgery or health centre, depending on where she is based. She will give you a phone number to get in touch if you need to.

Your family doctor (GP) can be contacted at any time for yourself, your baby or child. Many doctors will see small babies at the beginning of surgery hours or without an appointment if necessary, but be prepared to wait. Some will give advice over the phone.

Some GPs work closely with health visitors and run baby clinics and child health clinics (see below).

> You have to register your baby with your doctor. Do this as early as possible. When you register your baby's birth at the local registry office, you will be given a pink card with your baby's NHS number on it, to sign and take or send to your doctor. If you need the doctor to see your baby before you have registered the birth, you can go to the surgery and fill in a registration form for the doctor there.
>
> If you move, register with a new doctor close to you as soon as possible. (See page 86, 'How to change your GP'.)

Your child health clinic is staffed by health visitors and clinic doctors. You can talk to them about any problems to do with your baby or child. But if your child is ill and is likely to need treatment, you should go to your family doctor. Clinics offer regular health and development checks (see page 28) and immunisation (see page 59) for your baby or child. Many GPs also provide these services.

At many child health clinics you can get baby milk and vitamins cheaper than in the shops. If you are entitled to free baby milk and vitamins, or to low-price baby milk, you can get these at your clinic (see page 92, 'Help with national health services costs').

Clinics are good places to meet other parents. Some run mother and baby or parent and toddler groups. And there may be a noticeboard advertising local groups, secondhand baby clothes and equipment etc.

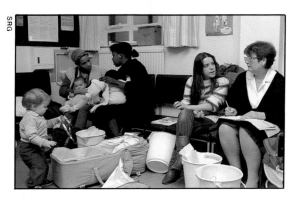

Your community health council (in your phone book under the name of your health authority) can advise you on how to get what you need from the health services and on what you are entitled to. It can also give you information about local services. For example, if you want to change your doctor, your CHC will have a list of local doctors and may know something about them.

Local authority services

Your social services department (in your phone book under the name of your local authority) can give you information about many of the local services for parents and children: day nurseries, childminders, playgroups, opportunity groups (which include children with special needs), family centres and so on. What is available varies from place to place – but it is always worth asking.

Many local authorities now produce booklets listing local services for families with under-fives. Ask at your local library, social services department, citizens advice bureau or other advice centre.

Social workers are usually based in social services departments. They can help with personal, practical and financial problems and can give information about local authority services in your area. They often also know a lot about voluntary organisations and local groups.

To contact a social worker, either about a particular problem or to get information about local services, phone your local social services department. Or ask your health visitor to put you in touch.

The housing department (in your phone book under the name of your local authority) is responsible for all council housing in your area and will run the council housing waiting list.

The housing department deals with applications for housing from people who are homeless. Under the law, they have a duty to house people in certain priority groups who are homeless (or are soon going to be) through no fault of their own. Priority groups include *pregnant* women and parents of children under 16.

Through your housing department, you should also be able to find out about local housing associations – which also provide housing for rent.

Your education department (in your phone book under the name of your local authority) is responsible for all the state-run nursery schools, nursery classes and infant schools in your area and can give you information about them.

The education department also has a responsibility to assess children with special needs and provide suitable education for them (see page 29).

Scotland and Northern Ireland

Community health council: In Scotland, community health councils are called local health councils. In Northern Ireland, they are called health and social services councils. Look in your phone book under the name of your local health board.

Social services department: In Scotland, the social services department is called the social work department (in your phone book under the name of your local regional council). In Northern Ireland, it is called the health and social services board (in your phone book under Health and Social Services Board).

Housing department: In Scotland, you will find your housing department in your phone book under the name of your local district council. In Northern Ireland, the housing department is called the housing executive (in the phone book under Housing Executive).

Education department: In Scotland, you will find your education department in your phone book under the name of your local regional council. In Northern Ireland, the education department is called the education and library board (in the phone book under Education and Library Board).

Where to go and who to go to

(There are many voluntary organisations which also offer help and support. See 'Finding other help' (page 87) and the list of organisations on pages 94-5.)

Health and medical problems

☐ Your community midwife, health visitor, child health clinic or family doctor.

Personal and family problems

☐ Your health visitor, family doctor or a social worker.

(See also 'Finding other help' on page 87.)

Benefits

(See pages 89-93 for information about social security benefits.)

☐ Your social security office (in the phone book under 'Social Security, Department of'; in Scotland, under 'Social Security, Department of; in Northern Ireland, under 'Government of Northern Ireland, Department of Health and Social Services).

☐ Your health visitor or a social worker.

☐ Your citizens advice bureau or other advice centre.

☐ Freeline Social Security – a telephone service, run by the Department of Social Security, giving information and advice on all social security benefits. The service cannot deal with individual claims, but can answer questions about benefits. Dial 0800 666555 (or in Northern Ireland 0800 616757). Your call is free of charge.

(Some voluntary organisations also offer advice on benefits. See pages 94-5.)

Housing

☐ Your local housing department.

☐ A social worker.

☐ Your citizens advice bureau or other advice centre.

☐ A local housing association. Your housing department should be able to put you in touch with housing associations in your area.

(Shelter is an organisation which offers information and advice on housing problems. Address on page 95.)

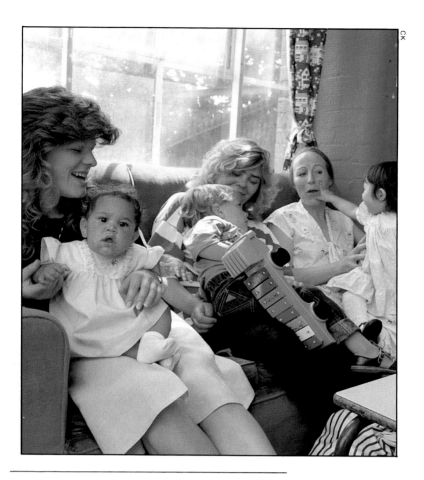

Child care and playgroups

☐ Your health visitor.

☐ Your social services department.

(You can also find out about playgroups through the Pre-school Playgroups Association – address on page 94.)

Nursery schools, nursery classes, infant schools

☐ Your local education department.

(Private nursery schools are not the responsibility of the local education authority but have to be registered with the social services department.)

Advice centres

Advice centres are any non-profit making agencies that give advice on benefits, housing and other problems. They include citizens advice bureaux, community law centres, welfare rights offices, housing aid centres, neighbourhood centres and community projects. Look for them under these names in your phone book, or under the name of your local authority.

Using the services

(A clinic doctor) **"I know the services often let parents down or don't give them what they need. All I can say is, parents have got to keep asking for what they want. If *they* don't do that, either for their children or for themselves, no-one else will."**

Around the country, the health and social services vary both in what they provide and in how well they provide it. Often it isn't easy to get what you want and need from the services.

The services are not the only source of help and support open to you (see 'Finding Other Help', opposite). But if you have, for example, a medical problem, you have no choice but to find medical help – and this will mean making the most of the services available.

○ Before you meet with any professional, try to get it clear in your mind exactly what you want to talk about and what information you can give that will be helpful. You may want to make some notes beforehand and take them with you as a reminder.

○ Unless your child needs to be with you, try to get a friend or neighbour to look after him or her so that you can concentrate. It's much easier to talk and listen if you are not distracted.

○ If you *do* have to go with your child/ children, take books or toys with you to entertain them.

○ Try to consider the answers or advice given to you. If your immediate feeling is 'but that wouldn't work for me' or 'that isn't what I'm looking for', then say so and try to talk about it. You're less likely to come away with an answer you're not happy with or can't put into practice.

○ If a problem is making life difficult or is really worrying you, it's worth pursuing it until you get some kind of answer, if not a solution. So if the first person you talk to can't help, ask if they can suggest where else you might go. Or if the doctor or health visitor suggests a remedy that doesn't work, go back and ask again.

○ Many professionals are not good at talking clearly and straightforwardly. So be determined and *ask* about anything you don't understand. Question jargon and medical terms, for example, and go back over what is said to you to get it straight.

○ If your first language isn't English, and/or there are cultural differences to overcome, talking with professionals and getting what you need from the services can be much more difficult. You may find you are given information or advice that's not just hard to understand but inappropriate as well.

In some areas, there are **linkworkers** or **health advocates** working within the health service who can help get over culture and language barriers. They can put parents' needs and anxieties across to professionals. Ask your health visitors if there is a linkworker or health advocate in your area.

How to change your GP

You may need to change your doctor if you move. You may want to change for other reasons, even if you are not moving house.

First find a GP who will accept you. See if anybody can recommend one. Your local CHC or family health services authority* (which used to be called family practitioner committee – see your medical card for the address) both keep a list of doctors in your area. You may have to try more than one GP before you find one willing to accept you, especially if you live in a heavily populated area. If you cannot find someone after several attempts, your FHSA will do it for you and you should send them your medical if you have it, or the name and address of your previous GP if not.*

When you call at the surgery of the doctor you have chosen, you may be asked why you want to change. You do not have to give a reason but if you do, try to avoid criticising your old doctor. Say something good about the new one instead. For example, the surgery may be easier to get to, the hours may be better, the doctor may have a good reputation for treating young children, the practice may be larger and provide more, or you may prefer a woman doctor, or a doctor who shares your cultural background.

Once you have found a doctor to accept you, leave your medical card with the receptionist. You do not have to contact your old doctor at all. If you have lost your medical card, your new doctor will probably ask you to complete a form instead, although sometimes you may be asked to contact the FHSA (in the phone book under the name of your heath authority), giving the name and address of your previous doctor, to obtain a medical card first. If you do not know your old doctor's name and address, this may take a while but if you need treatment in the meantime, you can approach any doctor who must take you on, at least temporarily. It is best to say from the beginning that you need treatment now if you are also asking to be permanently registered with that doctor.

*In Scotland, contact your local health board; in Northern Ireland get in touch with the Central Services Agency in Belfast.

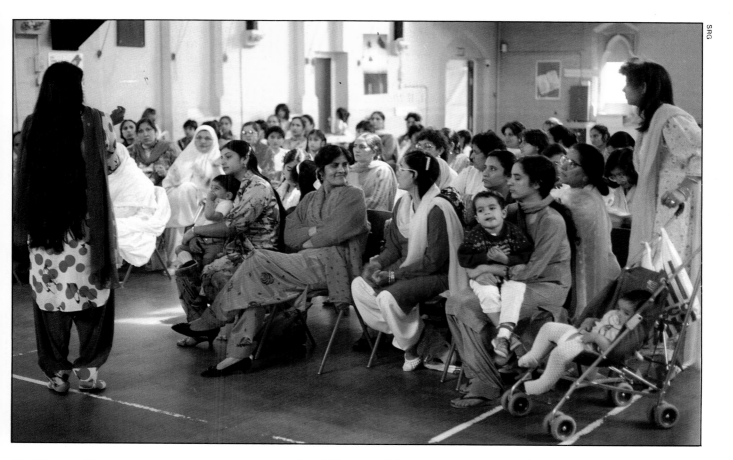

Finding other help

The help you want may not best come from the services or from professionals. There are many other sources of help available to parents – not only family and friends, but also many different kinds of local groups and voluntary organisations.

Local groups

To find out about local groups:

○ ask your health visitor or doctor

○ ask at your citizens advice bureau or other advice centre, your local library, your social services department, or your local Council for Voluntary Service (in your phone book, maybe as 'Voluntary Action Group', 'Rural Community Council' or 'Volunteer Bureau'). (In Northern Ireland, the Council for Voluntary Service is called the Council for Voluntary Action. In Scotland, contact the Scottish Council for Voluntary Organisations.)

○ look on noticeboards in your child health clinic, health centre, doctor's waiting room, local library, advice centres, supermarket, newsagent, toy shop . . .

○ look through the list of national organisations (page 94). Many run local groups.

○ In many areas there are now groups offering support to parents who share the same background and culture. Many of these are women's or mothers' groups. Your health visitor may know if there is such a group in your area. Or ask at places like your local library, your citizens advice bureau or other advice or community centre, your local Council for Voluntary Service, or your Community Relations Council (in your phone book, maybe as 'Council for Racial Equality' or 'Community Relations Office').

Making it happen

If you can't find a local group that suits you or can't find the support you need, think about setting it up for yourself. Many local groups have begun through a couple of mothers (say with crying babies, or sleepless toddlers, or just fed up and lonely) getting together and talking. You could advertise – on your clinic noticeboard, or in a newsagent's window or local newspaper. Or ask your health visitor to put you in touch with others in the same situation as yourself.

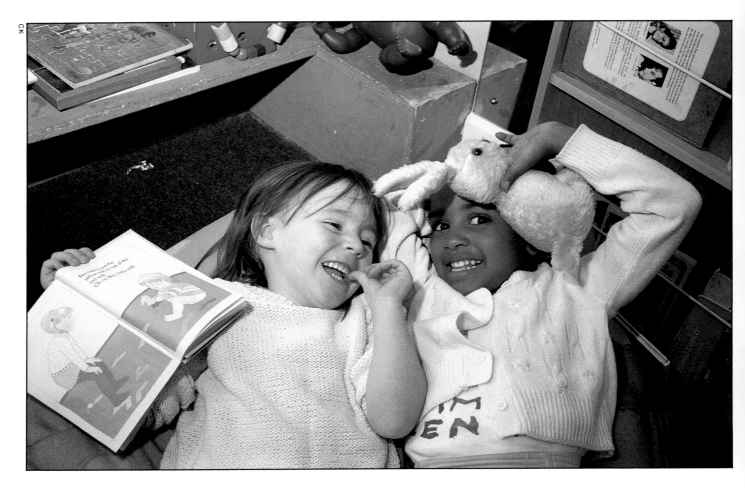

"I think looking after children is the hardest job going and the one you get least preparation for."

"The most important thing I do for them? Love them. I suppose sometimes they don't feel I love them – when I scream and shout. But I love them. And I try to show it."

"The thing is, you can't be perfect and the world's not perfect and they're not perfect either, no matter what you do. You can't change the world, and you can't change your children. You start off thinking you can control things, but you can't. You learn to accept a lot, being a parent."

"It took me a long, long time to get rid of the idea that every other mother in the world was a better mother than me. I think in the end it dawned on me that my own two children think I'm all right."

"The best thing is when they get to the age when they'll come to you and put their arms round you and give you a hug, just because they want to. That's the best feeling there is."

"Well, I'll never be the same, that's for sure. And I'd not have it any different."

Rights and Benefits

This is a guide to the main benefits available to families with young children. You may qualify for other benefits too. *It is always worth checking that you are claiming everything you are entitled to.* See the box below for where to go to get advice.

Government leaflets giving more information about particular benefits are listed under each benefit. You can get these leaflets

● from your local social security office
● from some large post offices
● from your citizens advice bureau or other advice centre
● by writing to the DSS Leaflets Unit, PO Box 21, Stanmore, Middlesex HA7 1AY.
● by phoning Freeline Social Security on 0800 666555 (or, in Northern Ireland 0800 616757).

The following leaflets give general information:

FB8 Babies and benefits A guide to benefits for expectant and new mothers.

FB27 Bringing up children? A guide to benefits for families with children.

FB28 Sick or Disabled? A guide to benefits if you're sick or disabled for a few days or more.

FB2 Which Benefit? A short guide to all social security benefits.

Rates of benefits are not given here as they change each year but you can find them in leaflet **NI196 Social security benefit rates.**

Where to get advice and help

Working out what benefits you are entitled to and making claims can be complicated. Get help if you need it.

● You can go to your social security office (in the phone book under 'Social Security, Department of'; in Scotland under 'Social Security, Department of'; in Northern Ireland under 'Social Security Agency'). Or go to your local citizens advice bureau or other advice centre (see page 85). Many social security offices are very busy and an advice centre is often the best place to go.

● A social worker should be able to advise you. Phone your social services department (social work department in Scotland, health and social services board in Northern Ireland — see page 84) and explain what help you want. Some local authorities also have welfare rights officers. Again, phone your social services department and ask.

● The Department of Social Security runs a free telephone service — Freeline Social Security. The service does not deal with claims but should be able to answer any questions about benefits. Dial 0800 666555 (or in Northern Ireland, 0800 616757).

● Some voluntary organisations offer information and advice on benefits. For example, the National Council for One Parent Families, the Scottish Council for Single Parents, the Maternity Alliance. See page 94 for details.

For parents

Child Benefit

This is a tax-free payment made to virtually anybody responsible for a child under 16. (You can also claim for a child aged between 16 and 19 who is in full-time education not above A level or an equivalent standard. In addition, Child Benefit may be extended for a few weeks for 16 and 17 year old school leavers who register for work or youth training.)

Child Benefit is paid —

● for each child you are responsible for. You don't have to be the parent to claim.

● every four weeks by a book of orders which you cash at the post office, or direct into most banks or building society accounts. If you are a one-parent family, or on Family Credit or Income Support (see page 91), you can choose to be paid weekly.

How to claim To claim Child Benefit for a new baby, use the coupon in leaflet **FB8 Babies and benefits** to get a claim form. Otherwise, ask for a claim form at your social security office. If you claim late, you can be paid in arrears for up to 6 months.
   If you're a couple (married or unmarried) the child's mother should claim. If a couple separates and live with other partners, one of the child's natural parents should claim.

Leaflets

FB27 Bringing up Children?
CH1 Child Benefit
CH4 Child Benefit for children away from home
CH5 Child Benefit for people entering Britain
CH6 Child Benefit for people leaving Britain.

One Parent Benefit

This is a tax-free addition to Child Benefit made to anybody bringing up a child on their own (whether or not they are the child's natural parent). You cannot claim if you are living with someone as husband or wife.

One Parent Benefit is paid —

● in line with Child Benefit (see above). It is paid in respect of the eldest dependent child and entitlement continues so long as you have a dependent child.

● with your Child Benefit, usually by a book of orders which you cash at the post office. You can choose to be paid weekly or every four weeks.

The amount paid is the same whatever your income or savings or however many children you have.

You cannot get One Parent Benefit if you are getting other benefits such as Widowed Mothers' Allowance, Guardians' Allowance or Invalid Care Allowance in respect of the same child.

One Parent Benefit does not affect Family Credit (see page 91), but any Income Support (see page 91) you get may be reduced by the amount of your One Parent Benefit.

How to claim Use the claim form in leaflet **CH11 One Parent Benefit**, or use the coupon in **FB8 Babies and benefits** to get a claim form.

If you have not yet claimed Child Benefit, claim it at the same time.

Leaflets
FB 27 Bringing up children?
CH11 One Parent Benefit
NP45 A guide to widow's benefits
NI14 Guardian's Allowance

New rights and benefits

This information applies to women whose babies are due on or after 16 October when new regulations for both maternity pay and leave come into force. All employed women will have a right to take 14 weeks' maternity leave and benefit rules will be changed. (NB If your baby is due before 16 October, you must have worked for two years full-time or five years part-time to qualify for the higher rate SMP and the right to return to your job. If you have worked for at least six months by the qualifying week, you will qualify for lower rate SMP. Check with your local DSS or the Maternity Alliance for details.)

Statutory Maternity Pay (SMP)

This is a payment for pregnant women in employment in the following circumstances.

● **If you have worked for the same employer for at least 26 weeks by the 15th week before the week your baby is due.**
You must have worked at least one day in the 15th week. If the 15th week is your twenty-sixth week of employment then you must work the whole week. To work out which is the 15th week before your baby is due, look on the calendar for the Sunday before (or on) which your baby is due. *Not* counting that Sunday, count back 15 Sundays. The 15th week before your baby is due begins on that Sunday. See the example on the calendar opposite.

and

● **Your average weekly earnings (normally the amount you have actually earned in the 19th to 26th weeks of your pregnancy) must have been at or above the amount where you start paying National Insurance contributions.**

SMP payments
● SMP is paid for 18 weeks. The first six weeks will be 90 per cent of your average weekly earnings, followed by 12 weeks at the lower rate of SMP.

● SMP is paid by your employer, either weekly or monthly, depending on how you're normally paid. Tax and National Insurance contributions may be deducted.

● You can choose when to start getting your SMP. The earliest you can start getting your SMP is 11 weeks before the week the baby is due. The latest date your maternity pay period can start is the week following the week in which you give birth, so you can work right up to the birth without losing any of your 18 weeks' maternity pay.

● SMP is paid regardless of whether you intend to return to work after your baby is born.

How to claim Write to your employer at least 21 days before you intend to stop work because of your pregnancy. Enclose your maternity certificate (**form MAT B1**), which is given to you by your doctor or midwife when you are about 26 weeks pregnant. If you don't get your maternity certificate in time, write to your employer anyway and send the form later. You may lose your right to SMP if you don't give 21 days' notice.
If you're unsure whether you can get SMP, ask your employer anyway. If you can't get SMP you may be able to claim Maternity Allowance (see opposite).

Leaflets
FB8 Babies and benefits
NI17A Maternity benefits (In Northern Ireland, **NIL17A**)

To get SMP you must have worked at least 1 day in this week

count back the weeks

Suppose this is the date your baby is due

Maternity Allowance

This is a benefit for pregnant women who have recently given up a job or who work but don't qualify for Statutory Maternity Pay (SMP) or who are self-employed.

You can claim it if –

● you are not entitled to SMP (see page 90) but have worked and paid standard rate National Insurance contributions for at least 26 of the 66 weeks ending in the week before your baby is due.

There will be two rates of MA –

● a lower rate, paid to self-employed women and those who have recently become unemployed.

● a higher rate, paid to women who are employed in the 15th week before the expected week of childbirth.

Maternity Allowance is paid –

● for up to 18 weeks, in the same way as SMP (See page 90). Payments start no earlier than 11 weeks before the week your baby is due.

● only for weeks when you are not working.

● by a book of orders that you cash at the post office.

When pregnant, and for a year after your baby is born, you can also get:

● Free NHS prescriptions. To claim during pregnancy, ask your doctor or midwife for form **FW8** as soon as you are sure you are pregnant. If you have had your baby and didn't claim while pregnant, use the claim form in **P11 NHS Prescriptions.**

● Free NHS dental treatment. To claim, simply tell your dentist that you are pregnant or have a baby under one year old.

You may also be able to get a Maternity Payment from the Social Fund (see page 93).

If you are on Income Support (see opposite), you can get free milk and vitamins while you are pregnant or have a child under 5.

How to claim Get form **MA1** from your antenatal clinic or social security office. Fill it in and send it to your social security office along with your maternity certificate (form **MAT B1**, given to you by your doctor or midwife when you are about 26 weeks pregnant). If you are claiming Maternity Allowance because you have been refused SMP, get form **SMP1** from your employer and send this with your claim.

Claim as early as possible after the start of the 14th week before your baby is due. If you have not paid 26 weeks' National Insurance contributions by this time, then you may decide to work later into your pregnancy and you should send off the **MA1** form as soon as you have made 26 National Insurance contributions. You may lose benefit if you claim after the birth.

If you have worked in the last couple of years and paid National Insurance contributions, it is worth claiming Maternity Allowance *even if you don't appear to qualify for it*. You may still be able to get Sickness Benefit if you have paid enough National Insurance contributions in earlier tax years. If you claim Maternity Allowance but don't qualify for it, you should automatically be considered for Sickness Benefit. Sickness Benefit is paid from the 6th week before the week the baby is due until two weeks after the baby is born.

Leaflets
FB8 Babies and benefits
NI17A Maternity benefits

For families

Family Credit

This is a tax-free benefit for working families with children.

It is not a loan and does not have to be paid back.

To be able to get Family Credit –

● you, or your partner, must be working at least 16 hours a week and

● you must have at least one child under 16 (or under 19 if in full-time education up to or including A-level or an equivalent standard).

You can qualify for Family Credit whether you are employed or self-employed, and whether you are a two-parent or one-parent family. (You may be single, married, or living with a partner as if you were married.) Your right to Family Credit does not depend on your National Insurance contributions.

Whether or not you get Family Credit, and how much you get, depends on you and your partner's net income, how many children you have and what age they are, what savings you and your partner have.

Family Credit is normally paid –

● for 26 weeks at a time. In each 26-week period, the amount you get stays the same, even if your earnings, or other circumstances, change during that time.

● weekly, by a book of orders which you cash at the post office, or if you prefer, every four weeks direct into your bank or building society account.

How to claim Use the **Family Credit Claim Pack FC1.** Fill in the claim form and send to the Family Credit Unit in the envelope provided.

If you get Family Credit, you can also get:
● free NHS prescriptions
● free NHS dental treatment
● NHS vouchers for glasses
● free travel to hospital for NHS treatment.

You may also be able to get payments from the Social Fund (see page 93). For example, a Maternity Payment to help buy things for a new baby.

If you have a child under one year old who is not being breast fed, you can get powdered baby milk at a reduced price. Take your Family Credit order book (or

notice of award of benefit if you are paid direct into your bank or building society account) to your local baby clinic to prove that you are getting Family Credit.

Leaflets
FC1 Family Credit Claim Pack
AB11 Help with NHS costs

Income Support

This is a benefit for anybody who does not have enough money to live on and has less than £8,000 in savings.

To be able to get Income Support –

● you must be aged 18 or over (or 16-17 if it is 11 weeks before your baby is due or if you have a child or face severe hardship) **and**

● you (or your partner if you have one) must be out of work or not working 16 hours or more a week.

How much Income Support you get depends on your age, whether you have a partner or dependants, your income, other benefits you are getting (such as Child Benefit or One Parent Benefit), and on how much you have in savings. Your right to Income Support does not depend on your National Insurance contributions.

Depending on your circumstances, Income Support payments can be made up of –

● a personal allowance for yourself and your partner (if you have one): and an allowance for any child or young person that you look after

● premium payments for people who have special expenses (such as families with children, lone parents, and parents of handicapped children – with disabilities.

● housing costs payments to cover certain costs, e.g. help with mortgage interest payments, not met by Housing Benefit (see page 92).

How to claim If you are unemployed, ask for an Income Support claim form at your unemployment benefit office (social security office in Northern Ireland). Anyone else should fill in the coupon in leaflet **IS1 Income Support**. If you send this coupon to your social security office, they will send you a detailed postal claim form for you to fill in.

If you get Income Support, you can also get:

● Housing Benefit (if you pay rent)
● Community Charge Benefit (see opposite)
● free NHS prescriptions
● free NHS dental treatment
● NHS vouchers for glasses
● free travel to hospital for NHS treatment (See 'Help with national health service costs', opposite).

If you get Income Support and are pregnant or have a child under 5, you can get tokens for free milk and vitamins. Ask your doctor or midwife for form **FW8** as soon as you are sure you are pregnant. Take or send it to your social security office. If you start getting Income Support only after your baby is born, claim your tokens on your Income Support claim form. If you have a baby under one year tokens can be exchanged for special baby milk or ordinary doorstep milk.

You may also be able to get payments from the Social Fund (see page 93). For example, a Maternity Payment to help buy things for a new baby.

Leaflets
AB11 Help with NHS costs
IS1 Income Support
SB20   A guide to Income Support
SB22   Income Support — new rules

Housing Benefit

Most people on Income Support and other people on low incomes can get help with their rent. You cannot get Housing Benefit if your savings are more than £16,000. If you pay rent to the council your Housing Benefit is paid direct to them and your bills will be smaller. If you pay rent to a private landlord your Housing Benefit is paid direct to you. If you are on Income Support you will usually get most or all of your rent (*not* including service charges) paid, but other low income families may get less depending on how many people are in the family, what their income is and how much the rent is. Your benefit will be reduced if you have more than £3,000 in savings. People on Income Support can claim Housing Benefit on form NHB1 when they claim Income Support. Get a form from your local council if you don't get Income Support.

Community Charge (poll tax) Benefit

This benefit helps people on Income Support or on a low income to pay their Community Charge. You cannot get Community Charge Benefit if your savings are more than £16,000.

People on Income Support can get a maximum Community Charge Benefit – 80% of the Community Charge in their area. For other low income families, how much benefit you get depends on your personal circumstances, for example, how many children you have and their ages, your income and savings, and the amount of Community Charge you have to pay.

People who claim Income Support can claim Community Charge Benefit at the same time on form **NHB1**. If you don't make a claim for Income Support get a form from your local council.

Help with national health service costs

All children under 16 automatically get:
● free NHS prescriptions
● free NHS dental treatment
● NHS vouchers for glasses.

Those under 19 and still in full-time education get free prescriptions, free dental treatment and vouchers for glasses. Those over 16 but not in full-time education get free dental treatment until they are 18.

All pregnant women and mothers of babies under one year old get:
● free NHS prescriptions
● free NHS dental treatment.

For how to claim, see 'For Pregnant Women', page 91.

If you get Family Credit or Income Support (see page 91), you automatically qualify for:
● free NHS prescriptions
● free NHS dental treatment
● NHS vouchers for glasses
● free travel to hospital for NHS treatment.

If you get Income Support and are pregnant or have a child under 5, you can also get tokens for free milk and vitamins. Look under 'Income Support' for how to claim.

If you get Family Credit and have a child under one year old, you can get baby milk at a reduced price. Look under 'Family Credit' for how to claim.

If you do not get Family Credit or Income Support but your income is low, you may still get some help with NHS costs. To find out if you qualify for help, get form **AG1 Help with NHS costs** (from hospitals, dentists and opticians as well as social security offices). Fill it in and send it to the Agency Benefits Unit in the pre-paid envelope provided with the form. (The Agency Benefits Unit does not exist in Northern Ireland: you should use your social security office.) The Unit will check your circumstances. If you qualify for help, you will be sent a certificate of entitlement, setting out the amount of help you can get for each type of charge. The certificate is valid for 6 months.

If your circumstances change, write to the Agency Benefits Unit – they will issue a fresh certificate if necessary.

Leaflets
AB11 Help with NHS costs
P11 NHS prescriptions
D11 NHS dental treatment
G11 NHS vouchers for glasses
H11 NHS hospital travel costs
WF11 NHS wigs and fabric support
FB28 Sick or disabled?

The Social Fund

The Social Fund offers help with certain expenses that are difficult to meet out of your regular income.

For example:

● If you are or your partner are getting Income Support or Family Credit (see page 91), you may be able to get a Maternity Payment to help buy things for a new baby. You can claim a Maternity Payment after the 29th week of pregnancy, up until the time your baby is 3 months old. If you are adopting a baby you can apply for Maternity Payment as long as the baby is not more than 12 months old when the application is made. The application must be made within three months of adoption. Any savings of over £500 will affect the amount of a Maternity Payment.

Get claim for **SF100** from an antenatal clinic or social security office.

● If you have a child under 5 years old and you are getting Income Support, you will automatically get a Cold Weather Payment for any consecutive 7-day period when the temperature averages 0 degrees Celsius or below. If you do not receive your payment, submit a written claim and ask for a written decision.

● If you are getting Income Support, you may be able to get a Community Care Grant. These non-repayable grants are given to help, for example, disabled people lead independent lives in the community. Sometimes grants are given to families under exceptional stress. Grants may be made for items such as furniture and house repairs. Any savings of over £500 will affect the amount of Community Care Grant.

Get form **SF300** from your social security office.

● If you have been getting Income Support for 26 weeks or more, you may be able to get a Budgeting Loan. These are interest-free loans made to help spread payment for certain expenses over a longer period. Loans may be made for items such as essential household equipment, safety equipment (such as a fireguard), furniture (such as bedding), repairs and maintenance.

The amount of the loan is decided by the Social Fund officer, according to your needs. The loan has to be repaid. Any savings of over £500 will affect the amount of a Budgeting Loan.

Get form **SF300** from your social security office.

● In an emergency, if you cannot afford something that is urgently needed, you may be able to get a Crisis Loan. These loans can cover living expenses for up to 14 days, or such things as essential household equipment or travel costs. Crisis Loans are only given if there is no other way of avoiding risk to somebody's health or safety.

. The amount of the loan is decided by the Social Fund officer. The loan has to be repaid.

For more information, contact a social security office.

Leaflets
SB16 A guide to the Social Fund

For children with special needs

If you have a disabled child who has needed a lot of extra looking after for at least three months, you may be able to get Disability Living Allowance. Leaflet **DLA1 Disability Living Allowance** gives more information and includes a claim form.

Income Support can be increased if you get Disability Living Allowance for a dependent child. Income Support is also increased if you receive Invalid Care Allowance.

If your child gets either the middle or the higher rate of the care component of Disability Living Allowance and you spend a lot of time looking after him or her, you may be able to get Invalid Care Allowance. You must be giving care for at least 35 hours a week and be earning less than a certain amount. **DS700 Invalid Care Allowance** claims pack tells you how to claim.

If your child has difficulty walking or needs supervision and guidance outside, you can claim the mobility component of Disability Living Allowance three months before his or her fifth birthday.

The **Family Fund** is a government fund, run independently by the Joseph Rowntree Foundation. It gives cash grants to families caring for very severely mentally or physically disabled children under 16. Grants are made to meet special needs not met by the health or social services – for example, a washing machine, special equipment, clothing, bedding, holiday expenses. Family income and circumstances are taken into account when applications are considered, but there is no means test. Write to the address on page 95 for more information and an application form.

This is only a brief guide to some of the benefits available. See page 89 for where to go for more information and for help with sorting out your entitlements and claims.

Useful organisations

Some of these organisations are large; many are small. Some organisations have local branches; some can put you in touch with local groups.

Where there are separate addresses for Scotland and Northern Ireland, these are given. If an organisation does not cover the UK, the area is indicated 'E' – England only 'E & W' – England and Wales 'NI' – Northern Ireland 'S' – Scotland

Organisations marked • produce publications. When you write, it is usually a good idea to send a large stamped addressed envelope for a reply.

Support and Information

Advisory Centre for Education (ACE) Ltd (E & W)
Unit 1B
Aberdeen Studios
22-24 Highbury Grove
London N5 2EA
(071) 354 8318 (Business line)
(071) 354 8321 (Advice line)
(Free advice line 2-5.00 Mon-Fri)
Independent education advice service for parents and children with special needs (see page 29).•

Alcohol Concern
Waterbridge House
32-36 Loman Street
London SE1 0EE
For information on local alcohol councils offering advice, information and support.•

The Association for Post-natal Illness (APNI)
25 Jerdan Place
London SW6 1BE
(071) 386 0868 (between 10 and 2)
Support for mothers suffering postnatal depression.•

Association of Breastfeeding Mothers (E & W)
Sydenham Green Health Centre
26 Holmshaw Close
London SE26 4TH
(081) 778 4769
24-hour telephone advice service for breastfeeding mothers. Local support groups.•

Community Health Councils
CHCs exist to help users of the national health service. They advise on where and how to get the service you need, and can help if you have a complaint.
In Scotland, CHCs are called local health councils; in Northern Ireland, health and social services. For your local CHC, look in your phone book under the name of your district health authority/health board.

Community Relations Councils (CRCs)
Commission for Racial Equality
10-12 Allington Street
London SW1E 5EH
(071) 828 7022
Sometimes called Councils for Racial Equality or Community Relations Offices. They are concerned with community relations in their area and often know of local ethnic minority organisations and support groups. To find your CRC, look in your phone book, ask at your town hall or local library, or contact the above.

CRY-SIS Support Group
BM CRY-SIS
London WC1N 3XX
(071) 404 5011
Help and support for parents of babies who cry excessively and/or sleep poorly.•

Enuresis Resource and Information Centre
Institute of Child Health
65 St Michael's Hill
Bristol BS2 8DZ
(0272) 264920
Provides advice and information to children, young adults, parents and professionals on bed-wetting.

Family Planning Information Service
27-35 Mortimer Street
London W1N 7RJ
(071) 636 7866
Information and advice on all aspects of family planning and contraception.•

Gingerbread
35 Wellington Street
London WC2E 7BN
(071) 240 0953
Self-help association for one-parent families. Local groups offer support, friendship, information, advice and practical help.

Home-Start Consultancy
2 Salisbury Road
Leicester LE1 7QR
(0533) 554988
A voluntary home-visiting scheme. Volunteers visit families with children under 5 and offer friendship, practical help and emotional support. Write for list of local schemes.

La Leche League (E, W & NI)
(Great Britain)
BM 3424
London WC1N 3XX
(071) 242 1278
Help and information for women who want to breast feed. Personal counselling. Local groups. Write with SAE for details of your nearest counsellor/group.•

Maternity Alliance
15 Britannia Street
London WC1X 9JP
(071) 837 1265
Information on all aspects of maternity care and rights. Advice on benefits, maternity rights at work.•

MAMA (Meet-a-Mum Association)
Cornerstone House
14 Willis Road
Croydon
Surrey CR0 2XX
(081) 665 0357
Support and help for women suffering postnatal depression, feeling isolated and tired after having a baby or just in need of a friend to share problems. Local groups and one-to-one contacts. Write with SAE for details of local groups.

National Association for Maternal & Child Welfare (NAMCW)
40/42 Osnaburgh Street
London NW1 3ND
(071) 383 4117
(071) 383 4541 (Education)
(071) 383 1315 (Publications)
Advice and courses on child care and family life.•

Action for Sick Children (NAWCH) (E)
Argyle House
29-31 Euston Road
London NW1 2SD
(071) 833 2041

Association for the Welfare of Children in Hospital (Wales)
Caroline Crimp
31 Penyrheol Drive
Sketty
Swansea SA2 9JT
(0792) 205 227

Action for Sick Children (NAWCH Scotland)
Mrs O Young
15 Smith's Place
Edinburgh EH6 8HT
(031) 553 6553
Support for sick children and their families – helping parents to be with their child in hospital and informing families about hospital care.•

NCT – The National Childbirth Trust
Alexandra House
Oldham Terrace
Acton
London W3 6NH
(081) 992 8637
(041) 633 5552 (Sales)
Help, support and advice for mothers, including breastfeeding information and support, antenatal classes, postnatal groups. Write for details of your nearest branch.•

National Council for One Parent Families
255 Kentish Town Road
London NW5 2LX
(071) 267 1361

One Plus
39 Hope Street
Glasgow G2 6AE
(041) 221 7150
Write or phone for free, confidential advice on pregnancy, housing, benefits, taxation, maintenance and other problems. Advice department closed Wednesdays.•

NSPCC (National Society for the Prevention of Cruelty to Children)
42 Curtain Road
London EC2A 3NH
(071) 825 2500
Aims to prevent all forms of child abuse. If you are in need of help, or know of anyone who needs help, look in the phone book for the number of your nearest NSPCC office.•

Parentline (E & W)
Westbury House
57 Hart Road
Thundersley
Essex SS7 3PD
(0268) 757007
Support for troubled parents in times of stress or crisis, chiefly through a confidential and anonymous telephone helpline.

Parents Anonymous
8 Manor Gardens
London N7 6LA
(071) 263 8918
A 24-hour telephone answering service for parents who feel they cannot cope or who feel they might abuse their children.

Parent Network (E & S)
44-46 Caversham Road
London NW5 2DS
(071) 485 8535
Runs 'Parent-link' groups, which offer a 'listening ear' and ideas on handling recurring daily situations that all parents face. Local support groups, newsletters and videos.

RELATE: Marriage Guidance
Herbert Gray College
Little Church Street
Rugby CV21 3AP
(0788) 573241
Confidential counselling on relationship problems of any kind. To find your local branch, look under RELATE or 'Marriage Guidance' in the phone book, or contact the above address.•

Twins and Multiple Births Association (TAMBA)
PO Box 30
Little Sutton
South Wirral L66 1TH
(051) 348 0020
Advice and support for parents of multiples. Network of local Twins Clubs.•

Women's Aid Federation (England)
PO Box 391
Bristol BS99 7WS
(0272) 633494 (administration)
(0272) 633542 (helpline)

Scottish Women's Aid
12 Torphichen Street
Edinburgh EH3 8JQ
(031) 221 0401
(between 10 and 1)

Welsh Women's Aid
2nd Floor
12 Cambrian Place
Aberystwyth
Dyfed SY23 1NT
(0970) 612748
38-48 Crwys Road
Cardiff
South Glamorgan CF2 4NN
(0222) 390874

Northern Irish Women's Aid
129 University Street
Belfast BT7 1HP
(0232) 249041
Provides refuge for women who have been sexually, mentally or physically abused. Information and practical help.

Women's Health
52 Featherstone Street
London EC1Y 8RT
(071) 251 6580
Information and support on many aspects of women's health. Provides a network of individual women who support others with similar health problems.•

Child Care / Play

National Childcare Campaign/Daycare Trust
Wesley House
4 Wild Court
London WC2B 5AU
(071) 405 5617/8
Campaigns for provision of good childcare facilities. The Daycare Trust gives information on finding child care, improving it, setting it up

National Childminding Association
8 Masons Hill
Bromley
Kent BR2 9EY
(081) 464 6164
An organisation for childminders, childcare workers, parents, and anyone with an interest in pre-school care. Works to improve status and conditions of childminders and standards of child care.•

Play Matters/The National Association of Toy and Leisure Libraries (E, W & S)
68 Churchway
London NW1 1LT
(071) 387 9592
Information about local toy libraries (which lend toys). For all families with babies and young children, including those with special needs. Runs ACTIVE groups which provide aids, information and workshops for disabled children.

Pre-school Playgroups Association
61-63 King's Cross Road
London WC1X 9LL
(071) 833 0991

Scottish Pre-school Playgroups Association
14 Elliot Place
Glasgow G3 8EP
(041) 221 4148

Northern Ireland Pre-school Playgroups Association
Unit 3
Enterprise House
Bouchar Crescent
Belfast
BT12 6HA
(0232) 662825
Help and advice on setting up and running parent and toddler groups and playgroups. Contact with local playgroups.

Mudiad Ysgolion Meithrin, The National Association of Welsh Medium Nursery Schools and Playgroups
10 Park Grove
Cardiff CF1 3BN
Advice and information on setting up and running Welsh language playgroups.

Working Mothers' Association
77 Holloway Road
London N7 8JZ
(071) 700 5771
Information and advice on childcare provision for working parents. Local groups.•

Working for Childcare
77 Holloway Road
London N7 8JZ
(071) 700 0281
Advice and information for employers, trade unions and others on workplace child care.•

Rights and Benefits / Money

(See also the Maternity Alliance and the National Council for One Parent Families, listed under 'Support and information'.)

Child Poverty Action Group
4th Floor
1-5 Bath Street
London EC1V 9PY
(071) 253 3406
Campaigns on behalf of low-income families. Provides advisors with information and advice for parents on benefits, housing, welfare rights etc.●

Citizens Advice Bureau
National Association of Citizens Advice Bureaux
115-123 Pentonville Road
London N1 9LZ
(071) 833 2181

Northern Ireland Headquarters
11 Upper Crescent
Belfast BT7 1NT
(0232) 231120

Citizens Advice Scotland
26 George Square
Edinburgh EH8 9LD
(031) 667 0156
For advice on benefits, housing, your rights generally and many other problems. To find your local CAB, look in the phone book, ask at your local library, or contact one of the head offices for the address. There may also be other advice centres in your area offering similar help.

Disability Alliance Educational & Research Association
Universal House
88-94 Wentworth Street
London E1 7SA
(071) 247 8776
Information and advice on benefits for all people with disabilities. Publish the *Disability Rights Handbook* – an annual guide to rights, benefits and services for those with disabilities and their families.

Family Fund
PO Box 50
York YO1 2ZX
(0904) 621115
A government fund independently administered by the Joseph Rowntree Memorial Trust. Gives cash grants to families caring for *very* severely handicapped children under 16. (See page 93.)

Housing

Shelter
88 Old Street
London EC1V 9HU
(071) 253 0202
Help for those who are homeless and advice on any kind of housing problem.●

Safety and First Aid

British Red Cross Society (BRCS)
9 Grosvenor Crescent
London SW1X 7EJ
(071) 235 5454

Scottish Red Cross Society
Alexandra House
204 Bath Street
Glasgow G2 4HL
(041) 332 9591
Among other activities, runs first aid courses through local branches. Look under British Red Cross or Red Cross in the phone book, or contact the above address.●

The Royal Society for the Prevention of Accidents (RoSPA)
Cannon House
The Priory Queensway
Birmingham B4 6BS
(021) 200 2461

RoSPA Scotland
Slateford House
53 Lanark Road
Edinburgh EH14 1TL
(031) 455 7457
Advice on the prevention of accidents of all kinds. Runs the Tufty Club for under-five year olds.●

St John Ambulance Association
1 Grosvenor Crescent
London SW1X 7EF
(071) 235 5231

St Andrew's Ambulance Association
48 Milton Street
Glasgow G4 0HR
(041) 332 4031
Runs local first aid courses. Look for your nearest branch in the phone book, or contact the above address.

Bereavement

Compassionate Friends
53 North Street
Bristol BS3 1EN
(0272) 539639
An organisation of and for bereaved parents. Advice and support. Local groups.●

The Foundation for the Study of Infant Deaths. (Cot Death Research and Support)
35 Belgrave Square
London SW1X 8QB
(071) 235 0965/1721
Support and information for parents bereaved by a sudden infant death.●

Stillbirth and Neonatal Death Society (SANDS)
28 Portland Place
London W1N 4DE
(071) 436 5881
Information and a national network of support groups for bereaved parents. Phone or write for details.●

Illness and Disability

AFASIC – Association for All Speech Impaired Children
347 Central Markets
Smithfield
London EC1A 9NH
(071) 236 3632/6487
Helps children with speech and language disorders. Information and advice for parents.●

Association for Spina Bifida and Hydrocephalus (ASBAH)
ASBAH House
42 Park Road
Peterborough PE1 2UQ
(0733) 555988

Scotland:
190 Queensferry Road
Edinburgh EH4 2BW
(031) 332 0743
Support for parents of children with spina bifida and/or hydrocephalus. Advice: practical and financial help. Local groups.●

Association of Parents of Vaccine Damaged Children
2 Church Street
Shipston-on-Stour
Warwicks CV36 4AP
(0608) 661595

Scotland:
Mrs H Scott
21 Saughton Mains Gardens
Edinburgh EH11 3QG
(031) 443 9287
Advises parents on claiming vaccine damage payment.

British Diabetic Association
10 Queen Anne Street
London W1M 0BD
(071) 323 1531
Information and support for all diabetics.●

Child Growth Foundation
2 Mayfield Avenue
Chiswick
London W4 1PW
(081) 994 7625
Information and advice for parents concerned about their child's growth.●

CLAPA – Cleft Lip and Palate Association
Dental Department
Hospital for Sick Children
Great Ormond Street
London WC1N 3JH
(071) 829 8614
Information and counselling for parents of newborn babies. Local groups.●

The Coeliac Society of the United Kingdom
PO Box 220
High Wycombe
Bucks HP11 2HY
(0494) 437278
(between 9.30 and 3)
Helps children diagnosed as having the coeliac condition or dermatitis herpetiformis.●

Contact a Family
170 Tottenham Court Road
London W1P 0HA
(071) 383 3555
Links families of children with special needs through contact lines. All disabilities. Local parent support groups.●

Cystic Fibrosis Research Trust
Alexandra House
5 Blyth Road
Bromley
Kent BR1 3RS
(081) 464 7211

Ireland: Mrs R Scott,
Anchor Lodge, Cultra, Co Down, N. Ireland.
(0232) 425 982

Scotland: Mr D Arthur
Inverallan
26 West Argyll Street
Helensborough
Dumbarton
G84 8DB
(0436) 676791

Wales: Mrs J Magness,
5 Ystrad Close, Johnstown, Carmarthen SA31 3PE
(0267) 237943
Support for parents of children with cystic fibrosis. Local groups.●

Disabled Living Foundation (DLF)
380-384 Harrow Road
London W9 2HU
(071) 289 6111

Disability Scotland
Princes House
5 Shandwick Place
Edinburgh EH2 4RG
(031) 229 8632

Disabled Living Centre
Musgrave Park Hospital
Stockman's Lane
Belfast BT9 7JB
(0232) 669501
Information and advice on all aspects of disability especially equipment and daily living problems. Referral to other organisations for disabled adults and children.●

Down's Syndrome Association (DSA)
155 Mitcham Road
Tooting
London SW17 9PG
(081) 682 4001

Scottish Down's Syndrome Association
158-160 Balgreen Road
Edinburgh EH11 3AU
(031) 313 4225

Northern Ireland Branch
2nd Floor
Bryson House
28 Bedford Street
Belfast BT2 7FE
(0232) 243266
Practical support, advice and information for parents of children with Down's syndrome.●

Haemophilia Society
123 Westminster Bridge Road
London SE1 7HR
(071) 928 2020
Information, advice and practical help for families affected by haemophilia.●

Hyperactive Children's Support Group
c/o Mrs S Bunday
71 Whyke Lane
Chichester
Sussex PO19 2LD
(0903) 725182 (9.30-3.30 Tuesday-Friday)
Information to help with problems related to hyperactivity and allergy.●

(I CAN) Invalid Children's Aid Nationwide (E & W)
Barbican City Gate
1-3 Dufferin St
London EC1
(071) 374 4422
Advice and information for parents of handicapped children, especially those with severe speech and language disorders.

MENCAP (Royal Society for Mentally Handicapped Children and Adults)
Mencap National Centre
123 Golden Lane
London EC1Y 0RT
(071) 454 0454

Scottish Society for the Mentally Handicapped
13 Elmbank Street
Glasgow G2 4Q4
(041) 226 4541
Information, support and advice for parents of mentally handicapped children. Local branches.●

Meningitis Research
Old Gloucester Road
Alverton
Bristol BS12 2LQ
(0454) 413344 (24 hours)
Meningitis Research provides updated information to the medical profession and advice, support and conselling to the general public through a 24-hour helpline.

MIND (National Association for Mental Health) (E & W)
Graata House
15-19 Broadway
Stratford
London E15 4BQ
(081) 519 2122
Help for people with mental illness. Also advice and information about coming off anti-depressants, tranquillisers etc. Local associations.

Muscular Dystrophy Group of Great Britain and Northern Ireland
7-11 Prescott Place
London SW4 6BS
(071) 720 8055
Support and advice through local branches and a network of Family Care Officers.●

The National Autistic Society
276 Willesden Lane
London NW2 5RB
(081) 451 1114

Scottish Society for Autistic Children
24D Barony Street
Edinburgh EH3 6NY
(031) 557 0474
Provides day and residential centres for the care and education of autistic children. Puts parents in touch with one another. Information and advice.●

National Deaf Children's Society (NDCS)
45 Hereford Road
London W2 5AH
(071) 229 9272

NDCS Technology Information Centre
4 Church Road
Birmingham B15 3TD
(021) 454 5151
(0800) 424 545 (freephone between 1 and 5)
Works for deaf children and their families. Information and advice on all aspects of childhood deafness. Local self-help groups.●

National Eczema Society (NES)
4 Tavistock Place
London WC1H 9RA
(071) 388 4097
Support and information for people with eczema and their families. Nationwide network of local contacts offering practical advice and support.●

National Meningitis Trust
Fern House
Bath Road
Stroud
Glos GL5 3TJ
(0453) 751 738
Information and support for those affected by meningitis. Local groups.

Positively Women
5 Sebastian Street
London EC1V 0HE
(071) 490 5515
Offers counselling and support services to women who are HIV positive.

Research Trust for Metabolic Diseases in Children (RTMDC)
Golden Gates Lodge
Weston Road
Crewe CW1 1XN
(0270) 250221 (office hours) or (0270) 626834, (0244) 881605
Makes grants and allowances for the medical treatment and care of children with metabolic diseases. Puts parents in touch with each other.

Royal Association for Disability and Rehabilitation (RADAR) (E&W)
12 City Forum
250 City Road
London EC1V 8AF
(071) 250 3222

Disability Action (NI)
2 Annadale Avenue
Belfast BT7 3UR
(0232) 491011
Information and advice on physical disability. Local organisations.●

Royal National Institute for the Blind (RNIB)
224 Great Portland Street
London W1N 6AA
(071) 388 1266
Information, advice and services for blind people.

SENSE, National Deaf-Blind and Rubella Association
11-13 Clifton Terrace
Finsbury Park
London N4 3SR
(071) 272 7774
Advice and support for families of deaf-blind and rubella handicapped children.

Sickle Cell Society
54 Station Road
Harlesden
London NW10 4UA
(081) 961 7795/8346
Information, advice and counselling for families affected by sickle cell disease or trait. Financial help when needed.●

Spastics Society
12 Park Crescent
London W1N 4EQ
(071) 636 5020

Scottish Council for Spastics
11 Ellersley Road
Edinburgh EH12 6HY
(031) 3135510

Northern Ireland for Orthopaedic Development (NICOD)
Malcolf Sinclair House
31 Ulsterville Avenue
Belfast BT9 7AS
(0232) 666188
Advice and support for parents of children with cerebral palsy.●

The UK Thalassaemia Society
107 Nightingale Lane
London N8 7QY
(081) 348 0437
Information, advice and support for families affected by thalassaemia.●

The Toxoplasmosis Trust
Room 26
61-71 Collier Street
London N1 9BE
(071) 713 0663
Information and advice for pregnant women and support and counselling for sufferers and their families.

Council for Disabled Children
8 Wakley Street
Islington
London EC1V 7QE
(071) 278 9441
Information for parents and details of all organisations offering help with particular handicaps.

Index